Ophthalmic Ultrasonography
and Ultrasound Biomicroscopy

Rasha Abbas

Ophthalmic Ultrasonography and Ultrasound Biomicroscopy

A Clinical Guide

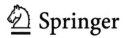

Rasha Abbas
Ultrasound Department
Watany Eye Hospital
Cairo, Egypt

ISBN 978-3-030-76981-9   ISBN 978-3-030-76979-6   (eBook)
https://doi.org/10.1007/978-3-030-76979-6

This Springer imprint is published by the registered company Springer Nature Switzerland AG
The registered company address is: Gewerbestrasse 11, 6330 Cham, Switzerland

Preface

This book is designed to help ophthalmologists better understand ocular sonography and its invaluable importance in the different fields of ophthalmology.

It offers a comprehensive guide with detailed information on the major aspects of ocular sonography, illustrated throughout with examples to provide the specialists with an overview on the different topics.

It is intended to give guidance on the basics of ocular sonography, as well as the key manifestations of different ocular diseases.

It is my hope and expectation that this book will provide effective learning experience and referenced resource for all ophthalmologists.

Cairo, Egypt   Rasha Abbas

Acknowledgments

Writing this book has been a surreal journey. It was both internally challenging and rewarding. I would like to take this opportunity to thank each individual who helped to make this happen.

First and foremost, I have to start by thanking my family for their ongoing support. This book would not have been possible without the endless patience and continuous encouragement of my lovely husband Ayman.

I'm indebted to Watany Eye Hospital team for supporting and giving me the opportunity to reach my goal.

I'm eternally grateful to my friends and colleagues for their insightful feedback and enthusiastic support. The support of the publisher and the collaboration of the editorial staff are warmly acknowledged.

I would like to express my appreciation and gratitude to the late Prof. Dr. Riyad Fikry, a special thanks to Prof. Dr. Nader Fathy, and lastly a heartfelt thanks to Marwa Faried and Dr. Samar sherif for their appreciated assistance.

Contents

Contributors

Sherif N. Embabi, M.D., Ph.D. Professer of Ophthalmology Ain Shams University, Vitreoretinal Consultant Watany Eye Hospital, Cairo, Egypt

Terese Kamal, M.D., FRCS Uveitis Consultant, Watany Eye Hospital, Cairo, Egypt

Fathy Fawzy Morkos, M.Sc., FRCS, FRCO. Professor of Ophthalmology in Military Medical Academy (Subspecialty: Anterior Segment Reconstruction, Cataract and Refractive Surgery), Chairman and Co-Founder of Watany Eye Hospital, Cairo, Egypt

Introduction and Ultrasound Examination

1

1.1 Physical Principles

Echoes: Echoes are produced by acoustic interfaces created at the junction of two media that have different acoustic impedance.

Acoustic impedance: The difference between the strength of the returning echoes from tissue boundaries with abrupt changes in acoustic properties. For example the anterior lens surface produces a stronger echo when bordered with aqueous than with hyphema because the difference between the lens and aqueous is greater than the difference in impedance between the lens and the blood.

Angle of incidence: The angle at which the sound beam strikes an interface is an important factor in the strength of the returning echoes. The more perpendicular the beam, the stronger is the returning echo.

Pulse echo system: The basic unit which includes a piezoelectric transducer to generate the ultrasonic wave, a receiver which processes the returning waves and a display screen.

Frequency: It is used in ophthalmic ultrasound ranging between 8–80 MHz [5, 10] compared to 2–6 MHz used in other fields of diagnostic ultrasound.

Resolution: The ability to distinguish between adjacent echoes, both axial(distance between two reflectors distinguishable from each other along the direction of acoustic propagation) and lateral (ability to distinguish the two reflectors positioned next to each other with respect to the ultrasound beam axis). This is enhanced by the use of a focused sound beam [6].

Gain: This is the procedure of increasing or decreasing the amplitude of echoes that are displayed on the screen.

© The Author(s), under exclusive license to Springer Nature Switzerland AG 2021
R. Abbas, *Ophthalmic Ultrasonography and Ultrasound Biomicroscopy*,
https://doi.org/10.1007/978-3-030-76979-6_1

Absorption: Ultrasound wave is absorbed by every medium through which it passes. The more dense the medium, the more absorption of the wave [2].

Display of signals: The received ultrasound signal can be displayed in three ways: A mode, B mode or a combination of both. Other modifications include the three-dimensional ultrasound, which uses a rotating transducer rather than the oscillating one used in the conventional ultrasound system and a combination of color Doppler with the B scan.

1.2   Instruments

A scan:

A-scan is a one-dimensional display of echo strength over time, There are two types of ultrasound A-scans: Biometric A-scan and standardized A-scan.

   Biometric A-scan: used primarily for axial length measurement, using a probe with 10–12 MHz and a linear amplification curve.

   Standardized A-scan: Pioneered by Ossoining, standardized A-scan was developed as a diagnostic tool in ophthalmology, It incorporate the S-shaped amplitude, which provide the benefit of the wide range of logarithmic amplification and the high sensitivity of linear amplification. Standardized A-scan utilizes an operating frequency of 8 MHz [1, 7, 8, 15].

B-scan:

B-scan is a two-dimensional brightness display, where the strength of the returning echo is displayed as a dot on the screen. The brightness intensity is proportional to the echo amplitude [6, 9, 11, 13, 18].

1.3   Clinical Application

1.3.1   Before Preforming B-Scan Examination

History taking and clinical examination of the eye are crucial initial steps before performing ophthalmic ultrasonography. History taking traditionally includes the presenting complaint, previous investigations or treatment related to the complaint, previous ocular surgeries, ocular traumas; as well as significant systemic illness and family history.

1.3.2 B-Scan Positioning and Examination

*Ultrasound examination is performed in the supine or sitting position.

*The probe is placed directly over the conjunctiva or cornea or placed over closed lids. The former has the advantage of reducing the sound attenuation caused by the lids; sterilization of the probe between procedures is mandatory [17].

*In cases of congenital anomalies and tumors, Examination of the other eye is mandatory.

*In cases of congenital anomalies, developmental glaucomas and trauma, comparing axial length measurements is recommended.

1.3.3 B-Scan Probe Orientation

The three basic probe orientation that are commonly used are axial, transverse and longitudinal scans.

A) Axial scan:

The Probe is directly applied to the cornea with the patient fixating in the primary gaze, The lens and optic nerve are displayed at the center of the scan.

In **Vertical** axial scan, the marker is placed in the superior position to examine the retina above and below the optic disc (Fig. 1.1).

In **Horizontal** axial scan, the marker is placed towards the patient nose which place the macular area below the optic disc (Fig. 1.2).

In **Oblique** axial scan, the marker is placed towards the upper of the two meridian examined (Fig. 1.3).

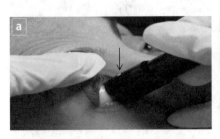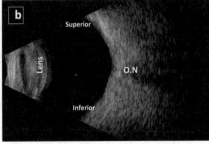

Fig. 1.1 Vertical axial B-scan, **a** the patient's eye in the primary gaze, and the probe is placed on the cornea, with the probe marker directed superiorly (black arrow), **b** B-scan showing the lens anteriorly and the optic nerve posteriorly with the upper part of the scan representing the superior portion of the globe (12 o'clock) and the lower part of the scan representing the inferior portion of the globe (6 o'clock). O.N: optic nerve

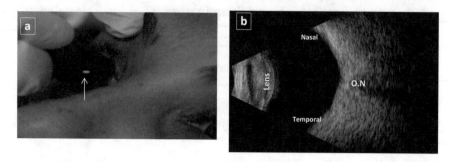

Fig. 1.2 Horizontal axial B-scan: **a** the patient's eye is in the primary gaze, the probe is placed on the cornea with the marker oriented nasally, **b** axial B-scan showing the lens anteriorly and the optic nerve posteriorly with the upper part of the scan representing the nasal portion of the globe (3 o'clock) and the lower part of the scan representing the temporal portion of the globe (9 o'clock)

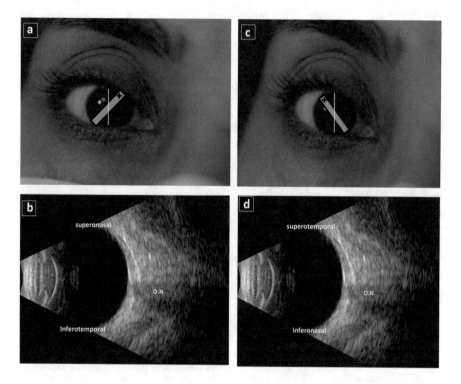

Fig. 1.3 **a** and **c** Schematic figure for oblique axial scan with the marker orientation superior, **b** and **d** B-Scan showing quadrants examined in oblique axial scan. O.N: optic nerve

B) Transverse Scans

In transvers scans, the probe is always placed parallel to the limbus demonstrating examination of the posterior fundus. To examine the fundus anterior to the equator, the patient is instructed to move his eye to the opposite direction of the probe.

*In **Vertical** transverse scan, the marker is directed upwards (Figs. 1.4 and 1.5).

*In **Horizontal** transverse scan, the marker is directed towards the nose of the patient (Fig. 1.6).

*In **Oblique** transverse scan, the marker is directed upwards.
   Transverse scans are used to show the lateral extent of a lesion.
   Example: To examine the nasal quadrant of the right eye, the probe is placed parallel to the limbus in the lateral quadrant, with the marker directed upwards, the resulted B-scan will represent a transverse scan of the 3 o'clock posterior to the equator. Shifting the probe away from the limbus (by instructing the patient to look to the opposite side of the probe) with the same probe orientation, the resulted B-scan will be a transverse scan of the 3 o'clock anterior to the equator (Figs. 1.4, 1.5 and 1.7).

C) Longitudinal Scans

The longitudinal scan probe orientation is perpendicular to the limbus where the marker is always directed towards the center of the cornea, to show the antero-posterior extent of a lesion.
   By placing the probe closer to the limbus the posterior fundus is easily examined; however, to examine the peripheral fundus the probe has to be moved towards the fornix.
   Example: To examine the 12 o'clock meridian, the probe is applied perpendicular to the limbus, with the marker directed towards the center of the cornea. The resulted B-scan represents a longitudinal view of 12 o'clock showing the fundus from the optic nerve to 12 o'clock posterior to the equator. By moving the probe towards the fornix, with keeping the same probe orientation, the resulted B-scan represents a longitudinal scan of 12 o'clock anterior to the equator and optic nerve will be displayed at the bottom of the scan (Figs. 1.8, 1.9, 1.10, and 1.11).

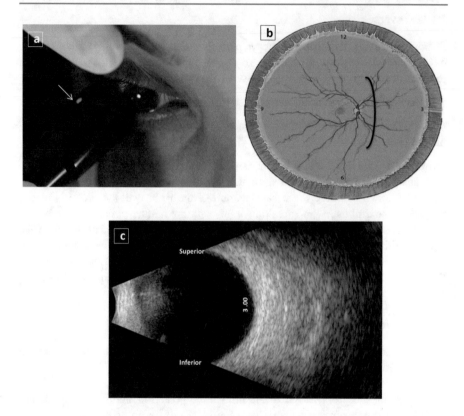

Fig. 1.4 Vertical transverse scan, **a** the probe is placed parallel to the limbus with the marker oriented superiorly (arrow) **b** schematic diagram showing the examined quadrant posterior to the equator **c** B-scan showing transverse scan of 3 o'clock meridian with the upper part of the scan representing the superior portion of the globe (12 o'clock) and the lower part of the scan representing the inferior portion of the globe (6 o'clock)

D) Examination of the Macula

Four basic probe positions that allow exposure of the macula.

*The horizontal axial scan (Fig. 1.12).

*The longitudinal scan (Fig. 1.13).

*The vertical transverse scan (Fig. 1.14).

*The vertical paraxial scan (Fig. 1.15).

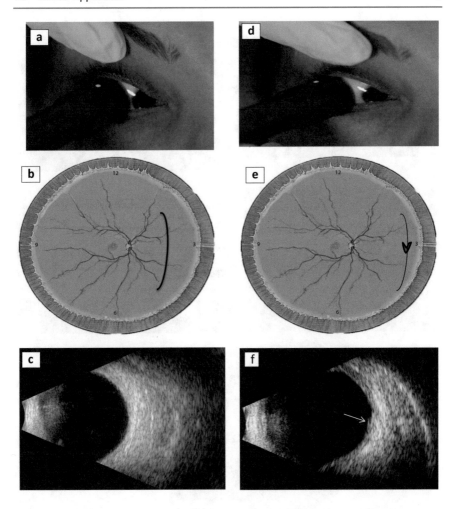

Fig. 1.5 Vertical transverse scan of 3 o'clock posterior to anterior aspect of the globe, (**a**) by asking the patient to fixate nasally, and by shifting the probe away from the limbus but not reaching the lateral angle (canthus) with the marker oriented superiorly, aiming for scanning 3 o'clock (around the equator as shown in the schematic diagram in (**b**) and with shifting the probe to the lateral canthus aiming to examine 3 o'clock anterior to the equator as shown in (**d** and **e**) (**c**) normal B-scan (**f**) B-scan showing the retinal break anterior to the equator

E) Paraxial Scan

The paraxial scan is used to examine the peripapillary area, It is similar to axial scan where the probe is placed over the cornea as in axial scan, then with the sound beam is slightly shifted so that the area of interest adjacent to the optic nerve is imaged (Fig. 1.15).

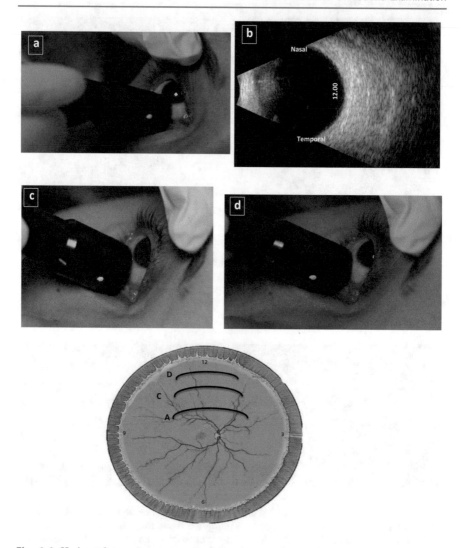

Fig. 1.6 Horizontal transverse scan examining the superior quadrant (12 o'clock) posterior reaching anterior aspect of the globe. **a** The patient is instructed to fixate superior and the probe placed parallel to the limbus with the marker oriented nasally. **b** B-scan of 12 o'clock posterior to the equator with the upper part of the scan representing 3 o'clock (nasal) and the lower part of the scan representing 9 o'clock (temporal), **c** and **d** showing the shift of the probe towards the inferior fornix to explore 12 o'clock, **c** around the equator, **d** anterior to the equator, **e** Schematic diagram demonstrating the examination of superior quadrant from posterior to anterior

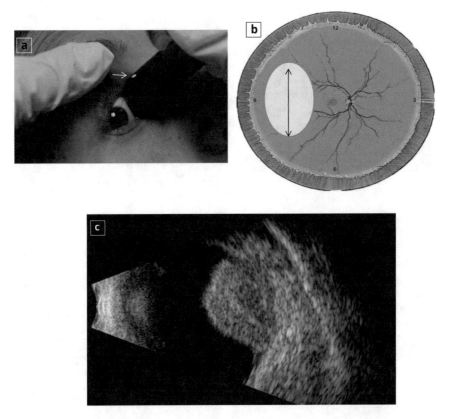

Fig. 1.7 Transverse scan of a lesion in the temporal quadrant, **a** the probe placed parallel to the limbus and shifted towards the medial canthus,with the marker oriented superior **b** schematic view of the lateral (circumferential)extent of the tumor (double arrow) **c** B-scan of a lesion in temporal quadrant for measuring the lateral extent of the lesion (crosser)

1.4 Diagnostic A-Scan:

Diagnostic A-scan is applied for quantitative evaluations of a tissue's structure, reflectivity and sound absorption [3, 4], and for kinetic evaluations of a tissue's vascularity, mobility and consistency.

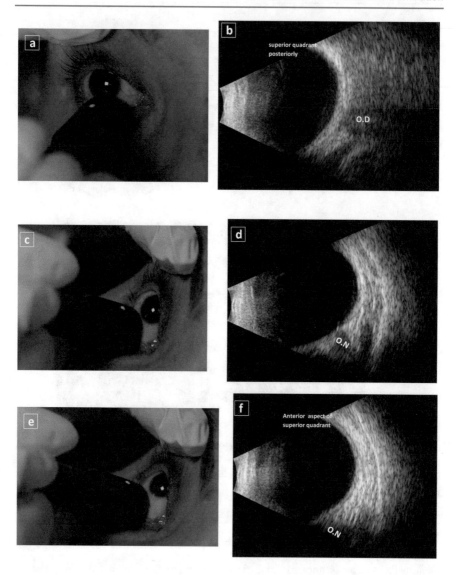

Fig. 1.8 Longitudinal scan of 12 o'clock, **a**, **c** and **e** the probe placed perpendicular to the limbus, with the marker oriented superiorly and the patient looking upward with shifting of the probe towards the inferior fornix to explore the anterior aspect of the globe at 12 o'clock. **b**, **d** and **f** B-scans showing the optic nerve shifted to the lower part of the scan to allow more exploration of the anterior aspect of the globe. O.N: optic nerve

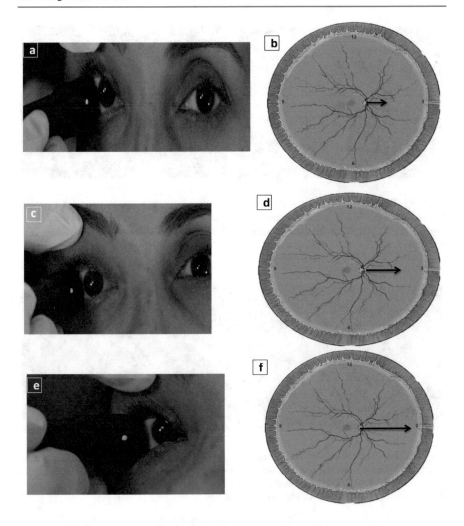

Fig. 1.9 Longitudinal scan of nasal quadrant at 3 o'clock, **a** the patient is in the primary gaze while placing the probe perpendicular to the limbus, and the marker directed towards the center of the cornea, **b** schematic diagram showing the posterior longitudinal scan of 3 o'clock posterior to the equator, **c** shifting the probe away from the limbus with the same probe orientation, **e** asking the patient to look more to the medial side to explore more of the anterior aspect of the globe at 3' o'clock, **d** and **f** schematic diagram demonstrating the examined longitudinal scans of 3 o'clock from posterior to anterior aspect of the globe

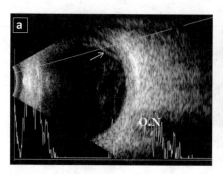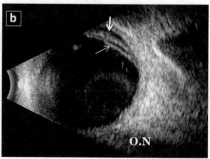

Fig. 1.10 Longitudinal scan, **a** peripheral retinal detachment with choroidal detachment (arrow), **b** anterior longitudinal scan to show the extend of the retinal detachment (thin arrow) with more exposure of the peripheral choroidal detachment (thick arrow) and the suprachoroidal space. O.N: optic nerve

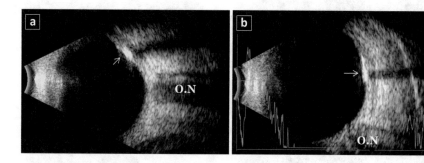

Fig. 1.11 Longitudinal scan of an osteoma, **a** osteoma in the nasal quadrant posteriorly, **b** anterior longitudinal scan for full exposure of the osteoma margin and to measure the anterior-posterior aspect of the lesion, as well as measuring the distance between the lesion and the optic disc for proper localization of the lesion. O.N: optic nerve

1.4.1   Quantitative Echography

1. Reflectivity:

The reflectivity is expressed by the height of the spike on A-scan (table) and the signal brightness on B-scan, where the sound beam must be perpendicular to the lesion being assessed.

Grade	low	Medium	Medium -high	High
A-scan height %	0–40	40–60	60–80	80–100

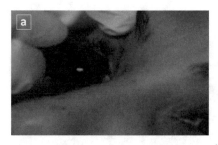
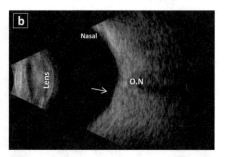

Fig. 1.12 **a** Horizontal axial view, with the patient's eye in the primary gaze, the probe placed to the cornea, and the marker oriented nasal, **b** B-scan of the macula just below the optic nerve (arrow)

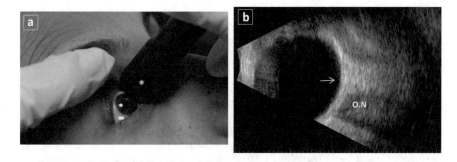

Fig. 1.13 **a** Longitudinal scan with the probe applied nasal and perpendicular to the limbus with the patient slightly fixating temporal, and the marker directed towards the center of the cornea, **b** longitudinal B-scan showing the macular area above the optic nerve (arrow). O.N: optic nerve

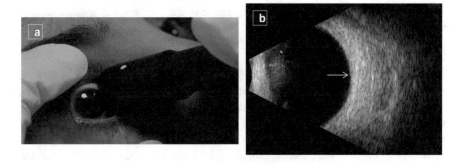

Fig. 1.14 Vertical transverse scan: **a** the patient is asked to slightly fixate temporal with the probe applied parallel to the limbus, and the marker directed superior **b** transverse B-scan showing the macula in the middle of the scan (arrow)

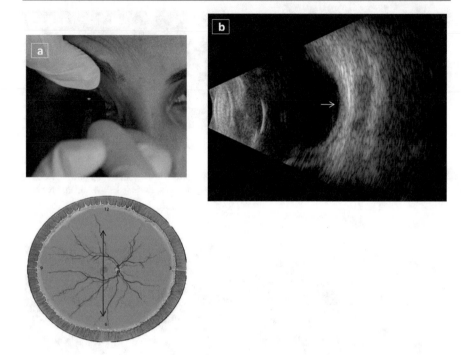

Fig. 1.15 Vertical Paraxial scan, **a** the patient fixates in the primary gaze with the probe placed on the cornea, and marker oriented superior with sound beam is shifted slightly to the peripapillary area (temporal to the disc) to examine the macula. Schematic diagram showing the examined part, **b** vertical paraxial B-scan showing the lens anteriorly and the macula posteriorly (arrow)

2. Internal Structure:

Internal structure refers to the degree of variations in histological architecture within a mass like lesion. A regular-homogeneous structure is represented by little or no variation in the height and length of the A-scan [9], while an irregular internal structure is represented with marked difference in the echographic appearance and with difference in the height and length of the A-scan (Figs. 1.16 and 1.17).

3. Sound Attenuation:

Sound attenuation or acoustic shadowing occurs when the sound energy is scattered, reflected or absorbed by a given media. It is seen on both A and B-scan [12].

In A-scan sound attenuation is indicated by progressive decrease in the height of spike and described as «kappa angle», If we draw a line from the peaks of the lesion spikes and direct it to the baseline(zero line), the angle formed between these two structures is the so-called «kappa angle». The steeper the angle the more sound attenuation will occur (Fig. 1.18b).

On B-scan, there is progressive decrease in strength of echoes or complete absence of echoes within or behind a lesion termed as shadowing [1] (Fig. 1.18).

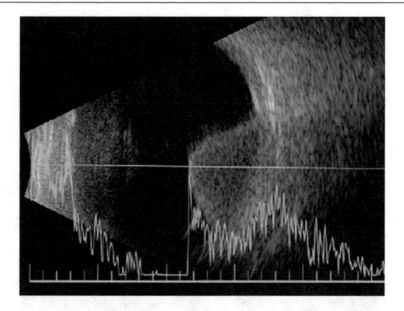

Fig. 1.16 A case of malignant melanoma with low and regular reflectivity on A-scan and low and homogenous echogenicity in B-scan

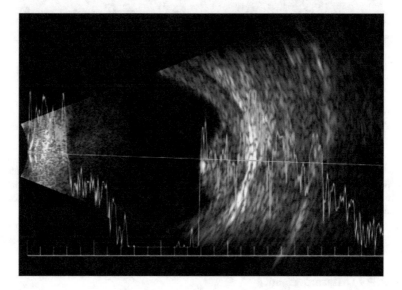

Fig. 1.17 a and **b** Scans of a lesion of irregular internal reflectivity on A-scan

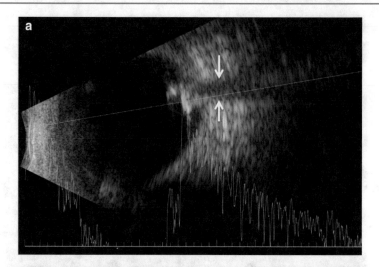

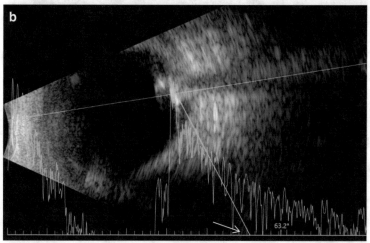

Fig. 1.18 **a** A case of foreign body impacted in the retina of high reflectivity followed by marked decrease in the height of the orbital spikes. Note the sound attenuation or shadowing behind the foreign body in B-scan (arrows), **b** measured angle kappa (arrow). Angle Kappa is proportional to the extent of sound attenuation, the greater the attenuation the greater the angle kappa

1.4.2   Kinetic Echography

1. Motility (Aftermovement):

Mobility or aftermovement of a membrane or vitreous opacity is produced when asking the patient to fixate on a target and the membrane or opacity in question is centered on the B-scan screen, then asking the patient to change their gaze direction and return back to the target. Vitreous detachment and retinal detachment exhibit an aftermovement.

2. Vascularity (Fast Spontaneous Motion):

Vascularity is characteristic of solid tumors, while the patient is examined in stationary position, vascularity is displayed as flickering of fast, low amplitude echoes on A-scan and B-scan.

3. Convection Movement (Slow Spontaneous Motion):

Convection movement is most commonly observed in longstanding hemorrhage, or layered inflammation or subretinal cholesterol as in Coat's disease. This movement is best assessed when the patient steadily fixates on a target while holding the probe stationary. Convection movement is slow, up and down motion of A-scan and a slow, circular motion on B-scan.

References

1. Ossoinig KC. Standardized echography: basic principles, clinical applications, and results. Int Ophthalmol Clin. 1979;19(4):127–210.
2. Lizzi FL, et al. Computer model of ultrasonic hyperthermia and ablation for ocular tumors using B-mode data. Ultrasound Med Biol Med Biol. 1992;18(1):59–73.
3. Thijssen JM, Bayer AL, Cloostermans MJTM. Computer-assisted echography: statistical analysis of A-mode video echograms obtained by tissue sampling. Med Biol Eng Compu. 1981;19(4):437–42.
4. Thijssen JM. Echo-ophthalmology: physical principles and diagnostic value. In: Photography, electro-ophthalmology and echo-ophthalmology in ophthalmic practice. Dordrecht, Springer; 1973. p. 273–318.
5. Coleman D, et al. Explaining the current role of high-frequency ultrasound in ophthalmic diagnosis. Expert Rev Ophthalmol. 2006;1(1):63–76.
6. Silverman RH. Focused ultrasound in ophthalmology. Clin Ophthalmol (Auckland, NZ). 2016;10:1865.
7. Hodes BL, Choromokos E. Standardized A-scan echographic diagnosis of choroidal malignant melanomas. Arch Ophthalmol. 1977;95(4):593–7.
8. Ossoinig KC, Frazier Byrne S, Weyer NJ. Part II: performance of standardized echography by the technician. Int Ophthalmol Clin. 1979;19(4):283–6.
9. Byrne SF. Standardized echography in the differentiation of orbital lesions. Surv Ophthalmol. 1984;29(3):226–8.
10. Pavlin CJ, Sherar MD, Stuart Foster F. Subsurface ultrasound microscopic imaging of the intact eye. Ophthalmology. 1990;97(2):244–50.
11. Baum G, Greenwood I. The application of ultrasonic locating techniques to ophthalmology: II. Ultrasonic slit lamp in the ultrasonic visualization of soft tissues. AMA Arch Ophthalmol. 1958;60(2):263–79.
12. Thijssen JM. The history of ultrasound techniques in ophthalmology. Ultrasound Med Biol. 1993;19(8):599–618.
13. Scott IU, et al. The impact of echography on evaluation and management of posterior segment disorders. Am J Ophthalmol. 2004;137(1):24–9.
14. Lizzi FL, et al. Ultrasonic spectrum analysis for tissue assays and therapy evaluation. Int J Imaging Syst Technol. 1997;8(1):3–10.

15. Henry MG, Hughes WF. Ultrasonics in ocular diagnosis. Am J Ophthalmol. 1956;41(3):488–98.
16. Dudea SM. Ultrasonography of the eye and orbit. Med Ultrason. 2011;13(2):171–4.
17. McLeod DAVID, Restori M. Ultrasonic examination in severe diabetic eye disease. Br J Ophthalmol. 1979;63(8):533–8.
18. Byrne SF. Ultrasound of the eye and orbit. Mosby Incorporated; 2002.

UBM Examination

2

2.1 Technique

Presently the probe used for UBM is small and light enough not to require a suspension arm. Scanning is performed with the patient in the supine position. A plastic eyecup of the appropriate size is inserted between the lids, holding methylcellulose or normal saline coupling medium (Fig. 2.1). To maximize the detection of the reflected signal, the transducer should be oriented so that the scanning ultrasound beam strikes the target surface perpendicularly [2]. The ultrasound probe is placed 2–3 mm from the ocular surface [7].

The transducer is not covered by a protective membrane such as that used with conventional ultrasound because of unacceptable sound attenuation from the membrane. The transducer is moving at a rate of 8 passes per second. Although the edges of the transducer are smooth, contact with the cornea could produce a corneal abrasion. An extra margin of safety is provided by the use of a soft contact lens on the cornea prior to examination to provide a barrier between the transducer and the cornea [5] (Fig. 2.2).

2.2 UBM Probe Positions

2.2.1 Axial Scan

The probe is immersed in the fluid bath perpendicular to the cornea over the pupil, allowing examination of two opposite quadrants. Axial UBM scanning allows the examination of the central thickness and transparency of the cornea, the depth and content of the anterior chamber, the position and pattern of the iris, the thickness, transparency and position of the lens, as well as the position of the intraocular lens [3, 4] (Figs. 2.3 and 2.4).

© The Author(s), under exclusive license to Springer Nature Switzerland AG 2021   19
R. Abbas, *Ophthalmic Ultrasonography and Ultrasound Biomicroscopy*,
https://doi.org/10.1007/978-3-030-76979-6_2

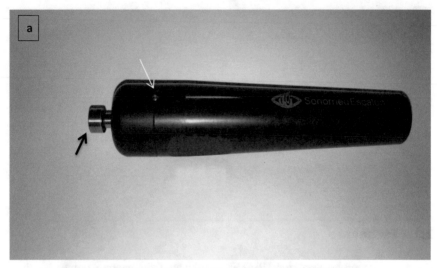

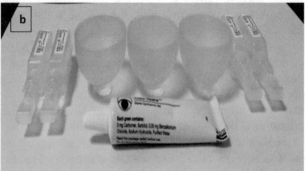

Fig. 2.1 **a** The UBM probe with the transducer attached to it (black arrow), the probe marker (white arrow). **b** Different sizes of eyecups, lubricant used to cover the cornea as well as sterilized fluid used as immersing fluid

2.2.2 Longitudinal Scan

The probe is applied perpendicular to the limbus with the marker directed towards the pupil according to meridian of interest. This UBM scan allow examination of the anterior chamber angle, the thickness, convexity and insertion of the iris, the thickness and structure of the ciliary body, the ciliary sulcus, the lens zonules and capsule, the haptics of the intraocular lens, as well as the peripheries of the vitreous and retina [3, 8]. Longitudinal scanning is used to measure the anterior to posterior extent of a lesion [4] (Fig. 2.5).

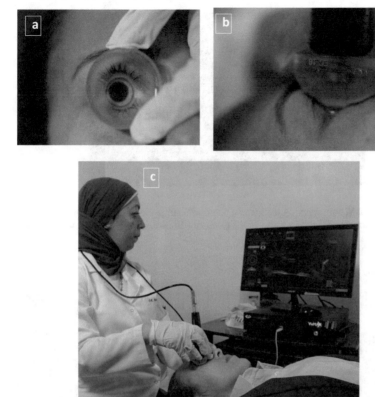

Fig. 2.2 a A fluid filled immersion eyecup applied to the eye, after applying topical anesthesia and lubricants to the cornea. **b** Application of the transducer inside the fluid filled eyecup. **c** The patient is lying down with the examiner seated behind the patient's head. The monitor is in an easily observed position, to facilatate observing the screen and the patient

2.2.3   Transverse Scan

The probe is applied parallel to the limbus over the central iris at the meridian of interest [3], the probe can be shifted towards the fornix to image peripheral iris, Ciliary body processes, pars plana and the peripheries of vitreous and retina (ora) [4, 8] (Fig. 2.6).

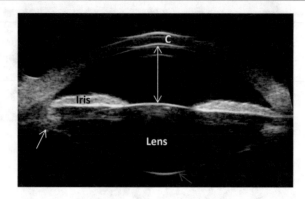

Fig. 2.3 Axial UBM scan showing the cornea, anterior chamber depth (double arrow) extending from the back of the cornea to the anterior lens capsule, the iris, the ciliary body (white arrow), lens with lens posterior capsule (red arrow)

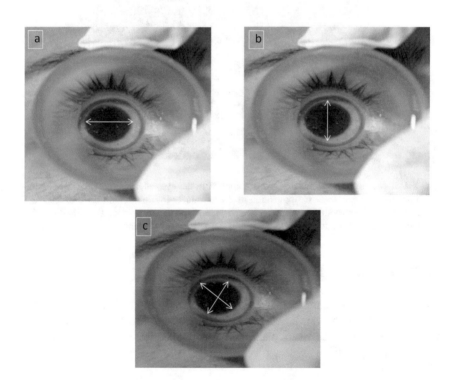

Fig. 2.4 Schematic diagram showing the quadrants examined in axial UBM, In figure **a** Horizontal axial UBM scan where 3 and 9 o'clock are examined from limbus to the opposite side **b** Vertical axial UBM scan to examine 12 and 6 o'clock **c** showing Oblique UBM scan

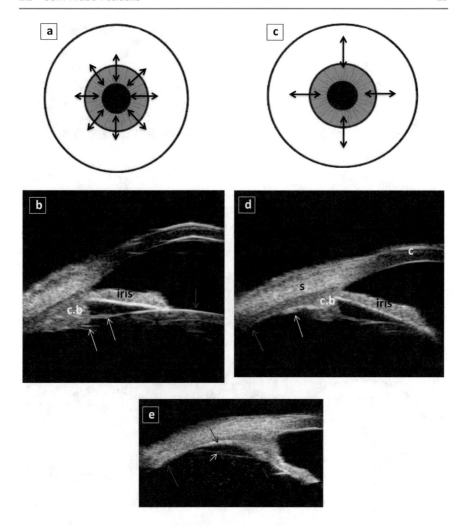

Fig. 2.5 a Schematic diagram showing how to examine different hours extending from the pupil to limbal area, with the probe applied perpendicular to the limbus with the marker directed towards the pupil **b** longitudinal UBM scan showing cornea, iris,angle, ciliary body, anterior lens capsule (red arrow), lens zonules (white arrows). **c** and **d** For Better visualization of the pars plana (white arrow) and peripheral retina (red arrow) by slight shifting of the probe away from the pupil. C:cornea S:sclera C.B: ciliary body. **e** longitudinal UBM scan showing the pars plana (black arrow) and anterior retina (red arrow) with multiple echoes and fine membranes in the anterior vitreous reaching the pars plana and anterior retina. Note the lens zonule (white arrow)

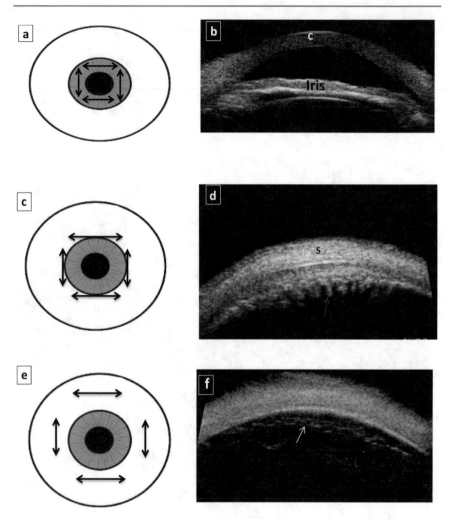

Fig. 2.6 **a** Schematic diagram showing the probe position parallel to the limbus over the central iris. **b** Transverse UBM scan showing the cornea and iris. **c** Schematic diagram showing the probe applied parallel and above the limbus. **d** Transverse UBM scan showing the ciliary body processes (red arrow). **e** Schematic diagram showing the probe applied parallel and shifted towards the fornix. **f** Transvese UBM scan showing the anterior retina with evidence of fine membrane in the anterior vitreous and over the anterior retina (white arrow)

2.3   The 10 Parameters Defined by Pavlin Et Al Which Are Commonly Used for Image Analysis of UBM [6] (Fig. 2.7)

1. The anterior chamber depth (ACD), measured from the corneal endothelium to the anterior lens surface.
2. The anterior chamber angle: this is the trabecular–iris angle measured with the apex in the iris recess and the arms of the angle passing through a point on the trabecular meshwork at 500 mm from the scleral spur and the point on the Iris perpendicularly opposite. Angle averaged 30(±11) degrees in our series of normal eyes.
3. The trabecular–ciliary process distance (TCPD), measured on a line extending from the corneal endothelium at 500 mm from the scleral spur perpendicularly through the iris to the ciliary process.
4. The angle opening distance 500 (AOD 500) (i.e., the distance between the posterior cornea surface and the anterior iris surface measured on a line perpendicular to the trabecular meshwork at 500 mm from the scleral spur) Results of measurement in normal cases was 347(±181) μm for AOD.
5. The iris distance 1 (ID 1) (i.e., the iris thickness measured along the same line as the TCPD) IDI (average thickness = 372 ± 58 μm).
6. The iris–ciliary process distance (ICPD): this is the "sulcus ciliaris" measured from the posterior iris surface (iris pigmented epithelium) to the ciliary process along the same line as the TCPD.
7. The iris–zonule distance (IZD): this corresponds to the posterior chamber depth measured from the posterior iris surface (iris pigmented epithelium) to the first visible zonular fiber at a point just clearing the ciliary process.
8. The iris–lens contact distance (ILCD), measured along the iris pigmented epithelium from the pupillary border to the point where the anterior lens surface leaves the iris.
9. The scleral– ciliary process angle (SCPA), measured between the tangent to the scleral surface and the axis of the ciliary process.
10. The scleral–iris angle (SIA), measured between the tangent to the scleral surface and the long axis of the iris.

Fig. 2.7 Pavlin's measurement parameters. (A) (AOD): The angle opening distance, (TIA, θ1): The trabecular—iris angle (B) (TCPD): trabecular ciliary process distance (ID1): Iris thickness is defined along this line, as is the iris –ciliary process distance (ICPD). (ID2): Iris thickness also can be measured 2 mm from the iris root (ID3): the iris at its thickest point near the margin (IZD):The iris—zonule distance. (ILCD): The length of iris—lens contact and the angle at which the iris leaves the lens surface (iris– lens angle; ILA, θ2) (PAVLIN, CHARLES J., KASIA HARASIEWICZ, and F. STUART FOSTER. Ultrasound Biomicroscopy of Anterior Segment Structures in Normal and Glaucomatous Eyes) [6]

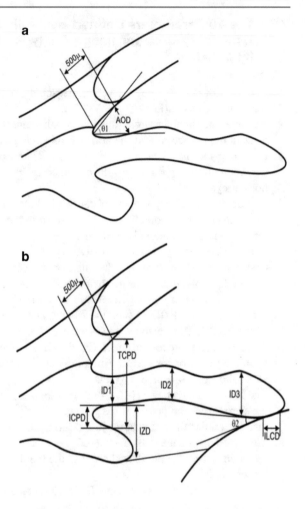

References

1. He M, Wang D, Jiang Y. Overview of ultrasound biomicroscopy. J Curr Glaucoma Pract. 2012;6(1):25.
2. Ishikawa H, Schuman JS. Anterior segment imaging: ultrasound biomicroscopy. Ophthalmol Clin North Am. 2004;17(1):7.
3. Ludwig K, et al. In vivo imaging of the human zonular apparatus with high-resolution ultrasound biomicroscopy. Graefes Arch Clin Exp Ophthalmol. 1999;237(5):361–71.
4. Pavlin CJ, Foster FS. Ultrasound biomicroscopy of the eye. Springer Science & Business Media;2012.
5. Singh AD, Lorek BH. Ophthalmic ultrasonography e-book: expert consult-online and print. Elsevier Health Sciences;2011.

6. Pavlin CJ, Harasiewicz K, Foster FS. Ultrasound biomicroscopy of anterior segment structures in normal and glaucomatous eyes. Am J Ophthalmol. 1992;113(4):381–9.
7. Byrne SF. Ultrasound of the eye and orbit. Mosby Incorporated;2002.
8. Gentile RC, et al. High-resolution ultrasound biomicroscopy of the pars plana and peripheral retina. Ophthalmology 1998;105(3):478–84.

Vitreoretinal Disease

3

3.1 Vitreous

The vitreous body is normally a homogeneous, optically, and acoustically transparent gel filling the posterior segment of the eye.

The volume of gel vitreous increases during the first decade of life, while the eye is growing in size and then remains stable until about the age of 40 years, when it begins to decrease in parallel with an increase in liquid vitreous [15].

*Conditions such as diabetes and myopia accelerate vitreous liquefaction and the formation of intravitreal collagen aggregates, which cause light scattering and can induce the clinical phenomenon of floaters.

Vitreous opacities produce dots or short lines on B-scan and vertical deflection from baseline on A-scan.

Opacities may originate from liquefied vitreous or clumps of cells, including calcium soaps (asteroid hyalosis), blood cells (haemorrhage), or inflammatory (uveitis) or infectious material (endophthalmitis).

3.1.1 Asteroid Hyalosis

Asteroid hyalosis is a benign degenerative condition of unclear pathogenesis that leads to the build-up of calcium phospholipid deposits within the vitreous, it is typically unilateral and asymptomatic [38].

Ophthalmoscopy reveals multiple yellow-white, iridescent opacifications of varied shape in the vitreous. Accordingly the condition was named for resembling **"stars on a clear night."** [1, 39].

© The Author(s), under exclusive license to Springer Nature Switzerland AG 2021   29
R. Abbas, *Ophthalmic Ultrasonography and Ultrasound Biomicroscopy*,
https://doi.org/10.1007/978-3-030-76979-6_3

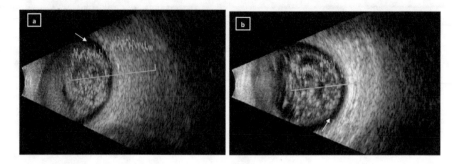

Fig. 3.1 Dense Astroid Hyalosis in different patients with multiple echoes of high amplitude in A-scan filling the vitreous cavity, note the clear vitreous space between the Astroid Hyalosis and the attached retina (white arrows)

The sonographic appearance shows multiple bright, point–like echoes of varying size, without causing acoustic shadowing. An area of clear vitreous is normally present behind the posterior boundary of asteroid hyalosis [3]. The A-scan of asteroid hyalosis is of medium to high reflectivity.

Movement of the eye resulted in significant after-movement of these opacities, giving the classic "**washing machine**" appearance as seen with vitreous hemorrhage [1], However, the sparkling appearance of the calcium phospholipid deposits in asteroid hyalosis differs from the duller heterogeneous echogenic layering shown with vitreous hemorrhage (Figs. 3.1, 3.2 and 3.3).

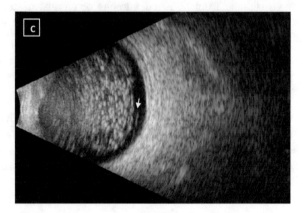

Fig. 3.2 Dense Asteroid hyalosis filling the vitreous cavity with partial posterior vitreous detachment (PVD), an area of clear vitreous behind the Asteroid hyalosis showing Partial PVD (white arrow)

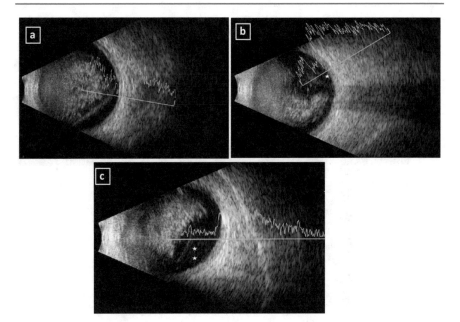

Fig. 3.3 A case of Asteroid Hyalosis **a)** Transverse scan showing multiple echoes of high amplitude filling the vitreous cavity (asteroid hyalosis) **b** and **c** with moving the eye in different position exposing the haemorrhage (stars) in the vitreous cavity of low to moderate amplitude in superimposed A-scan

3.1.2 Vitreous Hemorrhage

Vitreous hemorrhage is the second cause of opaque media after cataract, it occurs due to proliferative vascular retinopathies, trauma, disorders of coagulation, retinal breaks, polypoidal choroidal vasculopathy and tumors.

Ultrasonography is useful as a diagnostic, prognostic and follow-up tool, It helps to determine the source of vitreous haemorrhage and associated pathology [8, 9, 17, 18].

In Fresh mild haemorrhage: dots and short lines displayed on B-scan and low amplitude spikes on A-scan (Fig. 3.4).

In Dense haemorrhage: increase in the number of opacities with higher reflectivity

If organization of the blood occurs: A membranous surface will exist on B-scan with higher reflectivity on A-scan.

Gravity may cause the blood to layer inferiorly resulting in highly reflective pseudomembrane that can be confused with retinal detachment (the echogenecity of the pseudomembrane decrease superiorly and terminate in the vitreous gel) (Figs. 3.5 and 3.6).

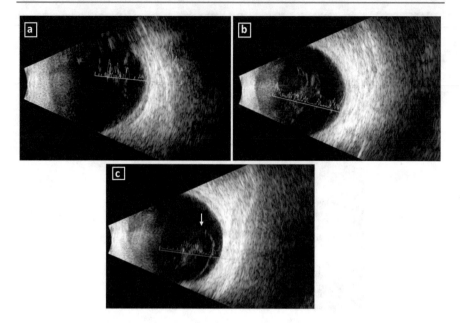

Fig. 3.4 Mild vitreous hemorrhage, **a** and **b** showing multiple echoes in the vitreous cavity of moderate amplitude in A-scan, with free mobility on kinetic scan, **c** Note the partial PVD) (arrow)

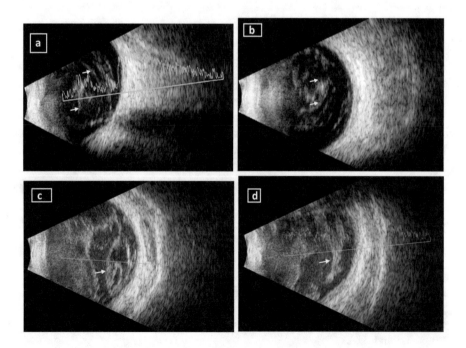

Fig. 3.5 Vitreous hemorrhage in different patients with different densities of the hemorrhage **a** and **b** showing moderate hemorrhage, **c** and **d** dense hemorrhage filling the vitreous cavity. with layering in all cases forming pseudomembranes (arrows)

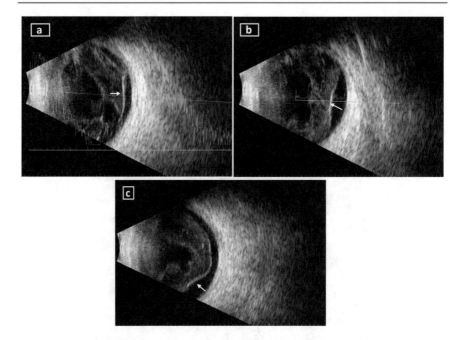

Fig. 3.6 Dense vitreous haemorrhage with thickened posterior hyaloid, **a, b** and **c** transverse scans of different quadrant of the eye demonstrating the thickened PVD (arrows)

3.1.3   Subhyaloid Hge

Subhyaloid haemorrhage can be present with or without vitreous haemorrhage, in B-scan it appears as echoes of low reflectivity, Therefore, a high gain is often needed. It is mobile even with longstanding cases (Figs. 3.7, 3.8 and 3.9).

Posterior Hyphema

Posterior hyphema is defined as dense haemorrhage in the subvitreal space where the cellular components of blood may settle and layer, the surface of this layered blood appear as dense membrane on B-scan with highly reflective spikes on A-scan simulating shallow localized retinal detachment (Figs. 3.10 and 3.11).

To differentiate it from localized retinal detachment

(A) Ask the patient moves his eye back and forth, the hyphema slides across the
     fundus surface.

     OR

(B) Ask the patient to sit upright or to turn his head. The hyphema will shift its
     position. It's important to hold the probe in the same position before and after
     the head/body is turned.

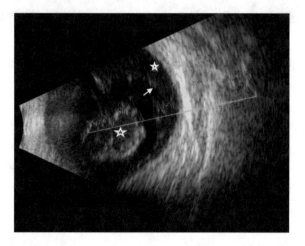

Fig. 3.7 A case of Vitreous hemorrhage (large star) with subvitreal hemorrhage, Note the PVD
(arrow) and the echoes in the subhyaloid space (small star), with low amplitude in the
superimposed A scan

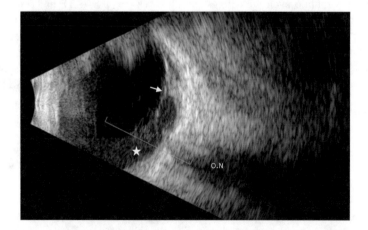

Fig. 3.8 A case of Subvitreal haemorrhage: multiple echoes in the subhyaloid space of low
echogenicity, with focal traction(arrow) on the retina temporal to the optic nerve (O.N: optic
nerve)

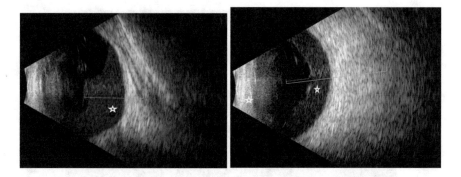

Fig. 3.9 Dense subvitreal haemorrhage in different patients, with multiple echoes of low echogenicity in the subvitreal space (stars)

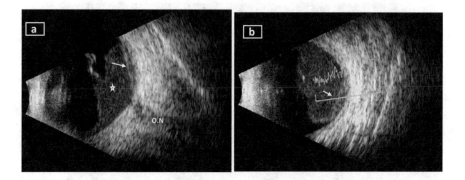

Fig. 3.10 Posterior hyphema: **a** Axial scan showing subvitreal hemorrhage with pseudomembrane (arrow) superior to the optic nerve (ON.), **b** the patient was asked to move his eye back and forth, the pseudomembrane (arrow) has shifted away from optic disc to the inferior quadrant

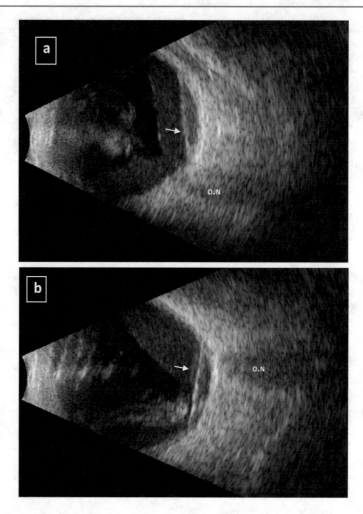

Fig. 3.11 Posterior hyphema:**a** Axial scan showing pseudmembrane superior to the optic nerve **b** The Patient was placed in the sitting position, note the pseudomembrane has shifted passing optic nerve to the inferior quadrant

3.2 Retina

One of the most important roles of ultrasound is to evaluate the status of the retina in the presence of opaque media. Retinal detachment have number of aetiology it can be either rhegmatogenous, tractional, combined traction-rhegmatogenous or exudative [31].

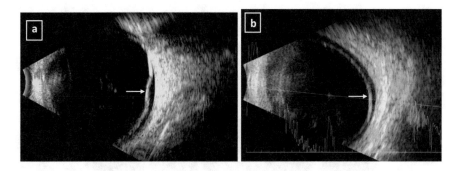

Fig. 3.12 Retinal detachment in two different patients, **a**, **b** retina (white arrows) appear as bright, smooth membrane, of high reflectivity on A-scan in (**b**)

Fig. 3.13 longitudinal scan showing bullous retinal detachment (arrow) in one quadrant, with high reflectivity on A-scan

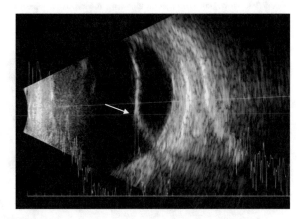

3.2.1 Rhegmatogenous Retinal Detachment

The detached retina appears as bright, continuous, somewhat folded membrane on B-scan. With high reflectivity on A-scan and the reflectivity remains equal along the extent of the membrane as long as the probe is perpendicular to it [26, 33].

Tethered, restricted after movements are seen in retinal detachment compared to a highly mobile posterior vitreous detachment. The mobility of the retina can vary depending on the duration of retinal detachment(R.D) and the presence of proliferative vitreoretinopathy(PVR) [41]

Configurations of the retinal detachment vary from shallow, flat and smooth to bullous and highly folded [19, 28] (Figs. 3.12, 3.13, 3.14, 3.15 and 3.16).

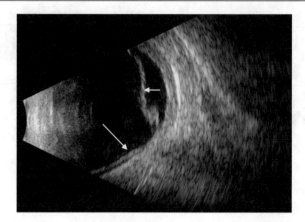

Fig. 3.14 Horizontal axial scan showing folded, more elevated retinal detachment (short arrow) in the temporal quadrant and smooth flat detachment (long arrow) in the nasal quadrant

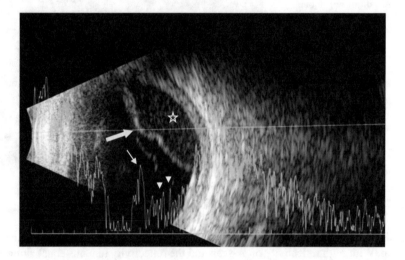

Fig. 3.15 Post-traumatic haemorrhagic retinal detachment: Transverse scan showing retinal detachment (thick arrow) with subretinal haemorrhage (star), A-scan with high reflectivity of the retina (thin arrow) and multiple irregular echoes of low to moderate amplitude (short arrows) of the subretinal haemorrhage

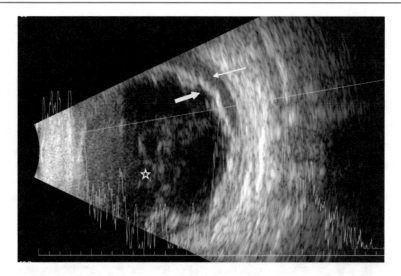

Fig. 3.16 Another case of retinal detachment with post-traumatic subretinal haemorrhage, Transverse scan showing retinal detachment(thick arrow)with high reflectivity in A-scan,, as well as multiple echoes in the subretinal space (subretinal haemorrhage) (thin arrow), Note the multiple and membranous echoes in the vitreous cavity consistent with vitreous haemorrhage (star)

3.2.2 Retinal Tears

A. Focal retinal tears

Focal retinal tears are a common cause of unexplained vitreous hemorrhage. It appears as small, focal, echo-dense membrane extending from the surface of the fundus to which the posterior hyaloid is attached. Kinetic echography is important in confirming the vitreoretinal adherence and the presence of retinal tear [7, 35] (Figs. 3.17 and 3.18).

Retinal tears are most commonly located along supratemporal and infratemporal retinal vascular arcade, and are located within 2 hours of the area of greatest elevation [6, 32, 36, 42].

Stalk like areas of neovascularization (as in Diabetic retinopathy or branch vein occlusion), small traction retinal detachment, focal accumulation of blood at area of vitreoretinal adherence, all those can simulate retinal tears [14] (Figs. 3.17 and 3.18).

B. Giant tear

B-scan of giant retinal tear appears as double linear echo connected to the optic nerve, the linear echo, which is not connected to the contour of the globe, represents the posterior flap of the giant tear inverted over the optic disc, the other linear echo

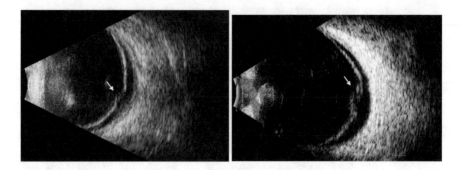

Fig. 3.17 Transverse scan in different patients showing retinal tears (white arrows) causing the retinal detachment

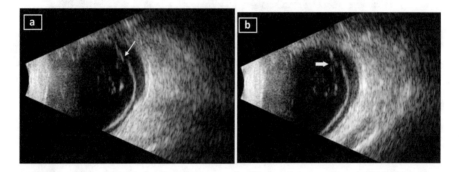

Fig. 3.18 a Longitudinal scan showing peripheral retinal tear (white arrows) causing shallow retinal detachment, **b** the posterior hyaloid attached to one edge of the tear (arrow)

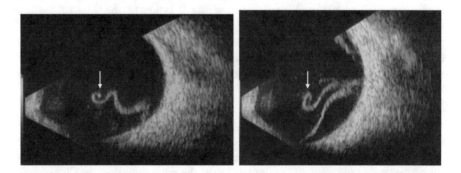

Fig. 3.19 Giant retinal tear, extensive folded retinal detachment with retraction and disinsertion from the periphery (arrow)

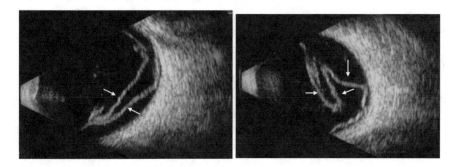

Fig. 3.20 The same patient with Giant retinal tear demonstrating the folded retinal leaves upon each other (arrows)

represent the detached retina. By moving the probe from midline towards the periphery of the fundus, the edge of the giant tear is reached and a single linear echo with both extremities connected to the orbital globe is seen (Figs. 3.19 and 3.20).

3.2.3 Traction Retinal Detachment

Traction retinal detachment is mainly caused by vitreous membranes or bands exerting traction on the retina causing retinal detachment. It is typically seen in diabetic retinopathy or trauma but can also occur in other conditions, (endophthalmitis, uveitis, retinopathy of prematurity and persistent fetal vasculature) [34]. Traction retinal detachment can be of mild or shallow, focal or frank retinal detachment.

Diabetic Retinopathy

Vitreoretinal adherence often occur in areas of proliferative preretinal membrane and stalks which are usually in the peripapillary region and around the vascular arcades, where traction retinal detachments are most commonly seen at these areas [27, 30]

Epiretinal membrane

Epiretinal membranes occur when new blood vessels, arising as a response to retinal ischaemia, penetrate the inner limiting lamina of the retina and grow within the cortical gel to form vascularised epiretinal membranes causing fibrous contraction within the epiretinal membrane and consequent tangential traction on the retina [4, 8, 10, 12].

The most common ultrasound retinal detachment configurations in diabetic retinopathy include:

(a) *Tentlike detachment*: produced by a point like vitreoretinal adherence (Fig. 3.21).

(b) *Table top detachment*: produced by a broader area of vitreoretinal adherence. Examination of the lesion with transverse and longitudinal view can differentiate between the tent-like and tabletop detachment (Fig. 3.22)

(c) *Hammock appearance*: when a posterior hyaloid form a bridge connecting closely spaced tent-like traction detachment (Figs. 3.23 and 3.24).

(d) *Ringlike or annular configuration*: peripheral retina traction secondry to anterior hyaloid fibrovascular, it typically occur following vitrectomy in phakic eyes. Anterior hyaloidal fibrovascular proliferation has been reported to be the most common severe complication after diabetic vitrectomy [24].

Other findings in diabetic retinopathy is macular oedema, characterized by mildly elevated dome shaped lesion with somewhat irregular surface contour with high to medium irregular reflectivity on A-scan. However, differential diagnosis of macular oedema includes AMD, inflammatory lesions of the retina as well as small tumours [11, 23] (Figs. 3.25 and 3.26).

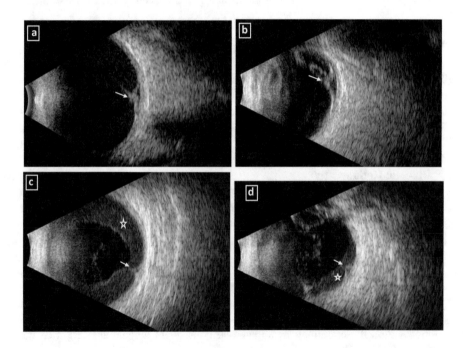

Fig. 3.21 Tent like traction retinal detachment. **a**, **b**, **c** and **d** Different patients showing variety of tent -like retinal detachment (arrows) caused by vitreoretinal adhesion, Note the subvitreal hge (stars) in (**c** and **d**)

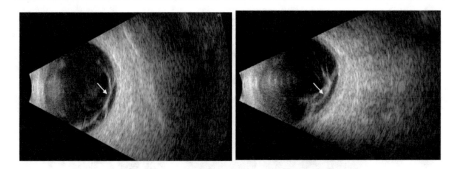

Fig. 3.22 Different patients with diabetic traction retinal detachment with broad area of vitreoretinal adherence producing table top configuration (arrows)

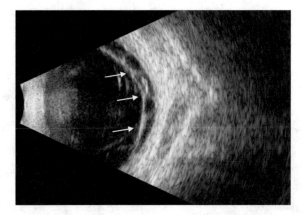

Fig. 3.23 Transverse scan of multiple traction retinal detachment (arrows) caused by bridging membrane posterior hyaloid (hammock appearance)

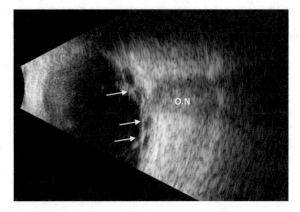

Fig. 3.24 Axial scan showing multiple focal traction retinal detachment around the optic disc, connected by bridging membrane posterior hyaloid (hammock appearance) Optic nerve (O.N)

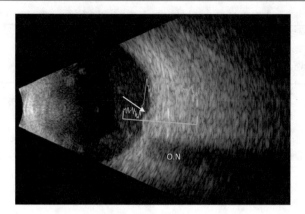

Fig. 3.25 Macular oedema: A longitudnal scan of the macula showing elevated dome shaped (arrow) with decreased internal reflectivity in the superimposed A-scan

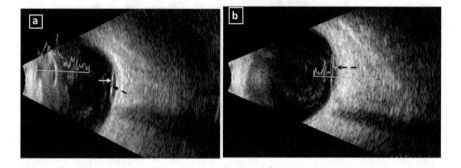

Fig. 3.26 A case with valsulva mannover, **a** Longitudinal scan showing hemorrhage (black arrow) elevating the internal limiting membrane(white arrow) of the macular area (which was confirmed by OCT), **b** Superimposed A-scan demonstrating the moderate amplitude of the internal limiting membrane followed by a decreased in amplitude due to the hemorrhage (black arrow) under the internal limiting membrane

3.2.4 Exudative Retinal Detachment

Exudative retinal detachment appears most commonly in uveal effusion, inflammation, central serous retinopathy and intraocular tumour. The ultrasound features include the presence of smooth bullae, and shifting fluid. The latter can be diagnosed by having the patient sit up or change head position which changes the configuration of the retinal detachment [50] (Figs. 3.27, 3.28 and 3.29).

Fig. 3.27 Exudative retinal detachment (thick arrow) due to malignant melanoma (dashed arrow). Showing subretinal echoes of low amplitude in A-scan (thin arrow)

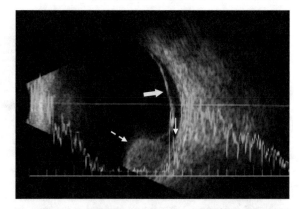

Fig. 3.28 A case of vitritis, echoes in the vitreous cavity collapsed anteriorly (Star) with exudative retinal detachment (thick arrow) echoes of low amplitude in the subretinal space (thin arrow)

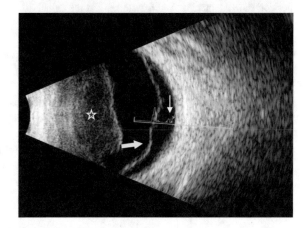

The presence of retinochoroidal thickening would indicate an inflammatory etiology such as scleritis, VKH or sympathetic ophthalmia [22, 51]. It is necessary to look for a tumor mass or granuloma if no break or inflammatory signs are noted.

3.2.5 Differential Diagnosis:

A) Retinal detachment (R.D) Versus Posterior vitreous detachment (PVD)

Retinal detachment can sometimes be confused with partial detachment of the posterior hyaloid face that is still attached to the disc. Differentiation can be difficult sometimes, therefore using additional technique may be useful [2, 5, 16, 37, 50]

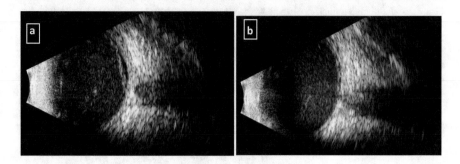

Fig. 3.29 Exudative retinal detachment: Two B scan images of the same patient demonstrating shifting fluid in an eye with an exudative retinal detachment. **a** the patient is placed in supine position showing retinal detachment temporal to the optic disc. **b** the patient is placed in sitting position showing that the fluid has shifted and the retinal detachment decreased

(a) The posterior insertion of the membrane in question should be carefully examined using all probe position, it can reveal an insertion of the membrane in the peripapillary area rather than the optic disc.

(b) Detection of another membrane anterior or posterior to the membrane in question, and finding the aetiology of the other membrane will facilities diagnosing the membrane in question.

(c) Using A-scan to follow the reflectivity of the membrane in question, In retinal detachment the A-scan will remain highly reflective, while in PVD the reflectivity will decrease when examining the peripheral fundus (Fig. 3.30).

B) Localized R.D and Retinoschisis

(a) Retinoschisis is a split in the outer plexiform layer, most often appears in the peripheral inferotemporal quadrant and usually bilateral.

(b) Retinoschisis appears as smooth, dome shaped,thin non mobile membrane in B-scan,with high reflectivity in A-scan which is smaller than that of retinal detachment [20] (Figs. 3.31, 3.32 and 3.33).

(c) For differentiation, apply scleral indentation during B-scan: In localized retinal detachment the space between the retina and the sclera will flatten as the subretinal fluid will escape through the break, while in retinoschisis the space narrow but doesn't flatten.

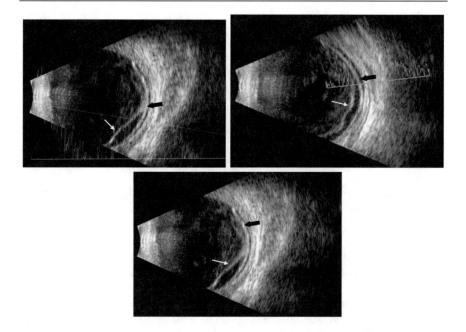

Fig. 3.30 PVD and R.D: Two membranes of high amplitude in A-scan, one of them representing a thickened posterior hyaloid (white arrow) and the other represent the retina (black arrow). In such cases all quadrants have to be examined closely for proper differentiation

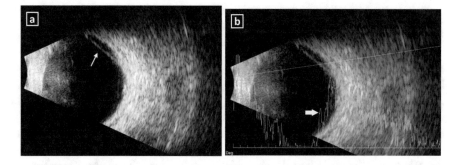

Fig. 3.31 Longitudinal scan of the right eye showing retinoschesis (arrow in **a**) in the inferotemporal quadrant anteriorly, smooth thin membrane immobile on kinetic scan, **b** showing the retinoschesis with lower echogenicity in B-scan than that of the detached retina, and with moderate to high reflectivity in A-scan

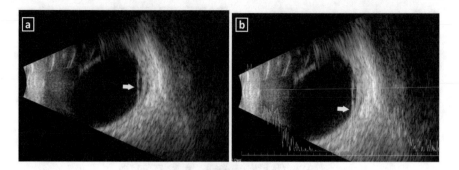

Fig. 3.32 Left eye of the same patient. Showing **a** retinoschisis in the inferotemporal quadrant, **b** with less reflectivity in A-scan compared to the detached retinal spike

3.2.6   Funnel Retinal Detachment: Long-standing Detachments

The retina is thickened and often shrinks to form a chord from the optic disc to the ora serrata, forming an intraocular triangle. The sides of the triangle represent stiff, highly detached retina, and the base of the triangle is an anterior bridging structure (proliferative vitreoretinopathy (PVR)) that connects the detached retina anteriorly [40] (Figs. 3.34, 3.35, and 3.36). Cyst-like structures of the retina in long-standing detachments are indicated ultrasonically by thickened and convoluted echo patterns [21] (Figs. 3.37, 3.38, 3.39 and 3.40).

3.3   Choroid

Retina, choroid and sclera (i.e posterior ocular wall) in the ultrasound appear as one layer of echo-dense in B-scan and as small group of highly reflective spike in A-scan.

Choroidal thickening can be focal or diffuse, which can be caused by oedema, inflammatory infiltration, tumour, choroidal folds [33]. In choroidal oedema, the retinochoroidal layer appears as thickened layer which can be distinguishable from the sclera on B-scan. Where in choroidal inflammation, the choroid appears as echolucent layer, with low to medium reflectivity on A-scan (Fig. 3.41).

3.3.1   Choroidal Detachment:

Choroidal detachment occurs when serous fluid or blood or inflammatory debris accumulates in the suprachoroidal space. In B-scan the suprachoroidal area appears as echolucent space in serous fluid accumulation [25, 43, 47], while in inflammatory

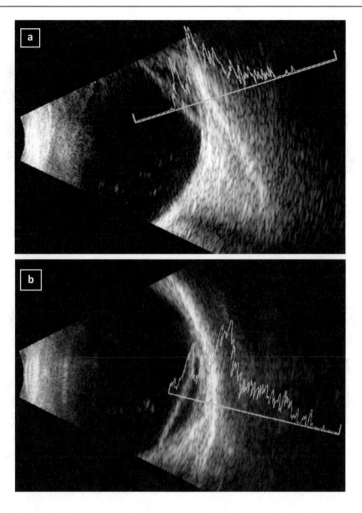

Fig. 3.33 Longitudinal scan (**a**) and transverse scan (**b**) localized retinal detachment showing thicker membrane with higher echogenicity in B-scan (compared to the retinoschesis), with high reflectivity in the superimposed A-scan

and haemorrhagic, appears as multiple dot-like in B-scan and of moderate to high reflective echoes in A-scan.

Typical choroidal detachment appears as smooth, thick, dome shaped membrane on B-scan and on A-scan shows a typical double peak or M-shaped spike which signify echoes from the choroid and the retina, However, shallow peripheral choroidal detachments appear as flat or concave instead of dome shaped [48]

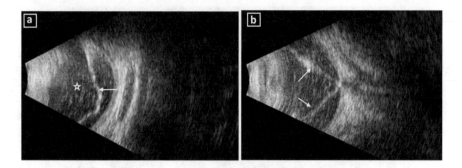

Fig. 3.34 Recurrent retinal detachment after silicone oil removal, **a** Transverse scan showing retinal detachment with hemorrhage in the vitreous cavity(star) and scattered echoes of high echogenicity (remnants of silicone oil) **b** Axial scan showing the open funnel retinal detachment (arrows)

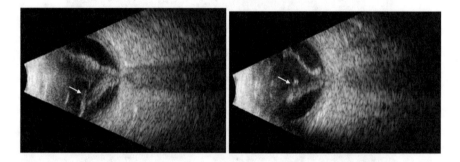

Fig. 3.35 Axial scans of different patients showing funnel shaped retinal detachment (open funnel) with thickened retinal leaves, with bridging membranes(arrow) indicating PVR and with limited mobility on kinetic scan

Peripheral choroidal detachment usually involve ciliary body (ciliochoroidal detachment) [44], or it can extended posteriorly 360 degree. In some cases of 360 degree choroidal detachment, the highly elevated choroidal detachment cause an apposition of the temporal and nasal detachment (kissing or appositional choroidal detachment). A fine bands stretching from the inner surface of the detached choroid to the sclera may be observed in B-scan, representing the vortex vein (Figs. 3.42, 3.43, 3.44, 3.45, 3.46, 3.47, 3.48 and 3.49).

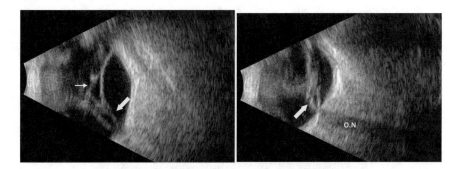

Fig. 3.36 Longitudinal scans of different patients showing funnel shaped retinal detachment. The funnel near the optic disc is almost closing (thick arrow) with thickened retinal leaves and bridging membranes (thin arrow) denoting PVR, with limited mobility on kinetic scan. (Optic nerve: O.N)

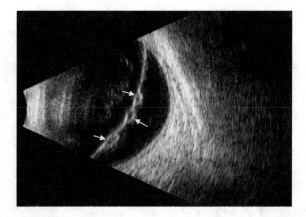

Fig. 3.37 A case of old retinal detachment, transverse scan of multiple retinal cysts (arrows) with limited mobility on kinetic scan

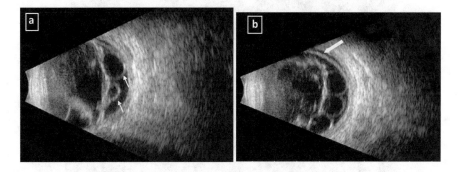

Fig. 3.38 A case of old retinal detachment **a** longitudinal scan showing retinal detachment with thickened retinal leaves with multiple large retinal cysts (arrows) **b** longitudinal scan exposing the periphery with evidence of choroidal detachment anteriorly(arrow)

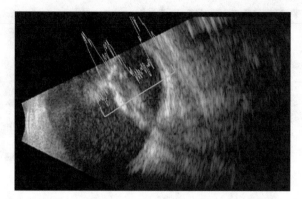

Fig. 3.39 Closed funnel retinal detachment, longitudinal scan showing a tightly closed funnel retinal detachment with thickened retinal leaves (indicating PVR), with high amplitude in A-scan

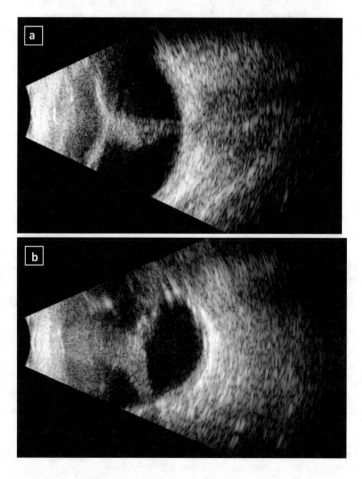

Fig. 3.40 Closed funnel retinal detachment **a** axial scan **b** longitudinal scan showing a T-shape tightly closed funnel retinal detachment, indicating PVR

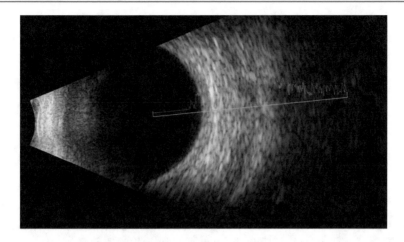

Fig. 3.41 Retinochoroidal thickening, which can be distinguishable from the sclera, with high internal reflectivity in the superimposed A-scan

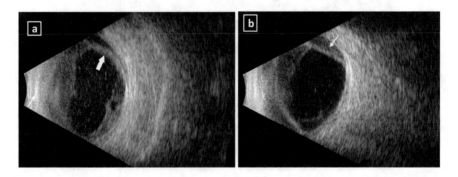

Fig. 3.42 Longitudinal scans showing peripheral ciliochoroidal detachment (thick arrow in **a**) with haemorrhage in the suprachoroidal space (thin arrow in **b**)

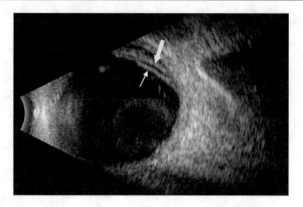

Fig. 3.43 Longitudnal scan showing peripheral ciliochoroidal detachment (thick arrow) with shallow retinal detachment (thin arrow) and echolucent suprachoroidal space

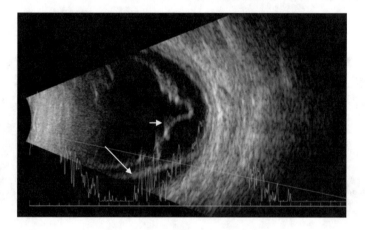

Fig. 3.44 Transverse scan showing retinal detachment (small arrow) with peripheral choroidal detachment (long arrow) with echolucent suprachoroidal space

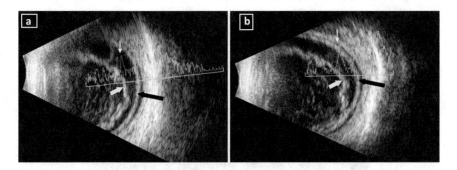

Fig. 3.45 Flattened globe with decreased axial length compared to the patient's fellow eye, **a** longitudinal **b** transverse scans showing retinal detachment with corrugated appearance (thick white arrows)with high reflectivity on A-scan(white thin arrow), and shallow choroidal detachment (black arrows)

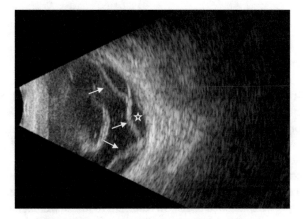

Fig. 3.46 Multiple dome-shaped choroidal detachment (arrows) with multiple echoes in the superachoroidal space (star)

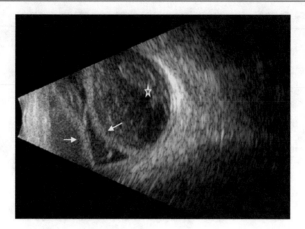

Fig. 3.47 Oppositional choroidal detachment (arrows) with haemorrhage in the suprachoroidal space (star)

3.4 Intraocular Silicone

Sound velocity of silicone oil is much slower than that of normal ocular tissue. Therefore, echogram of silicone filled eyes appear much larger than normal in supine position. Although techniques for detecting retinal detachment in eyes with silicone oil have been reported, experience indicates that ultrasound is not always reliable to detect retinal detachment .

In prone position due to movement of silicone oil towards the retina, a single spike corresponding to the scleral spike merging with the posterior oil surface was observed in cases with attached retina. In recurrent retinal detachments revealed two separate spikes despite the patient being in prone position [29] (Figs. 3.50, 3.51, 3.52 and 3.53).

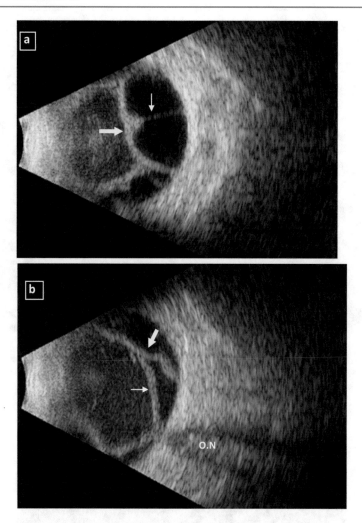

Fig. 3.48 **a** Peripheral bullous choroidal detachment(thick arrow) with a band- like in the suprachoroidal space representing a vortex vein (thin arrow), **b** longitudnal scan showing retinal detachment central (thin arrow) and choroidal detachment (thick arrow).(optic nerve: O.N)

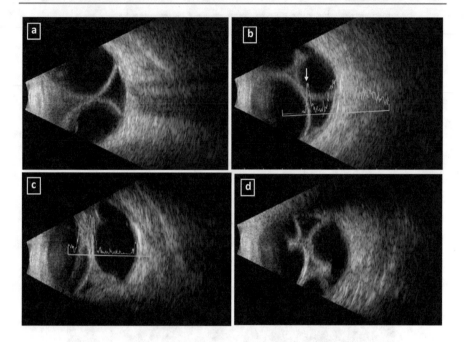

Fig. 3.49 Bullous choroidal detachment **a** Axial scan showing kissing choroid **b** Transverse scan with the superimposed A-scan showing the M-shaped spike(arrow) (C&D) longitudinal scans of the kissing choroid exposing the choroidal detachment anteriorly

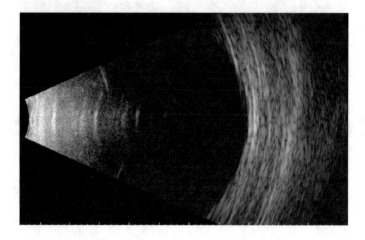

Fig. 3.50 Silicone filled eyes appear much larger than normal eye in supine position

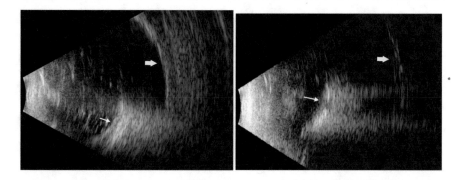

Fig. 3.51 Different patients with silicone filled eye, the patients are examined in the prone position to be able to scan the normal ocular wall, The retina in both patients are attached in the examined quadrants. Note the difference between the normal ocular wall (thin arrow) and the elongated axial length produced by the injected silicone oil (thick arrow)

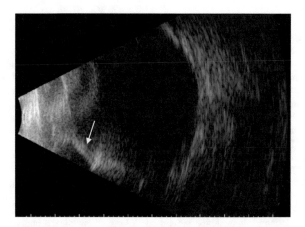

Fig. 3.52 Silicone filled eye with Patient examined in the prone position showing recurrent retinal detachment (arrow)

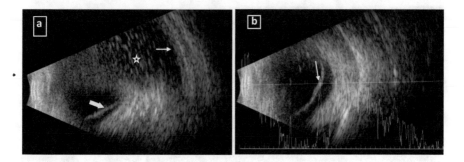

Fig. 3.53 Silicone filled eye while the patient is examined in prone position **a** showing recurrent retinal detachment in the examined quadrant (thick arrow) and the elongated axial length produced by the injected silicone oil(thin arrow), with multiple echoes in the vitreous cavity due to emulsified silicone oil (star). **b** Exposing more of the retina which is facilitated by the presence of emulsified silicone with high reflectivity of the retina in A-scan (arrow)

References

1. Stringer CEA, Ahn JS, Kim DJ. Asteroid hyalosis: a mimic of vitreous hemorrhage on point of care ultrasound. Can J Emerg Med. 2017;19(4):317–20.
2. Rabinowitz R, et al. Comparison between clinical and ultrasound findings in patients with vitreous hemorrhage. Eye. 2004;18(3):253–6.
3. Yamaguchi T, et al. Detecting vitreomacular adhesions in eyes with asteroid hyalosis with triamcinolone acetonide. Graefe's Arch Clin Exp Ophthalmol. 2007;245(2):305–8.
4. Mohamed IE, et al. Use of ophthalmic B-scan ultrasonography in determining the causes of low vision in patients with diabetic retinopathy. Eur J Radiol Open 2018;5:79–86.
5. Ivastinovic D, et al. Evolution of early changes at the vitreoretinal interface after cataract surgery determined by optical coherence tomography and ultrasonography. Am J Ophthalmol. 2012;153(4):705–9.
6. Sarrafizadeh R, et al. Incidence of retinal detachment and visual outcome in eyes presenting with posterior vitreous separation and dense fundus-obscuring vitreous hemorrhage. Ophthalmology 2001;108(12):2273–8.
7. Carrero JL. Incomplete posterior vitreous detachment: prevalence and clinical relevance. Am J Ophthalmol. 2012;153(3):497–503.
8. Capeans C et al. Ocular echography in the prognosis of vitreous haemorrhage in type II diabetes mellitus. Int Ophthalmol. 1997;21(5):269–75.
9. Tilanus MAD, et al. Relationship between anticoagulant medication and massive intraocular hemorrhage in age-related macular degeneration. Graefe's Arch Clin Exp Ophthalmol. 2000;238(6):482–5.
10. Tagawa H, McMeel JW, Trempe CL. Role of the vitreous in diabetic retinopathy: II. Active and inactive vitreous changes. Ophthalmology 1986;93(9):1188–92.
11. De Maeyer K, et al. Sub-inner limiting membrane haemorrhage: causes and treatment with vitrectomy. Br J Ophthalmol. 2007;91(7):869–72.
12. McLeod DAVID, Restori M. Ultrasonic examination in severe diabetic eye disease. Br J Ophthalmol. 1979;63(8):533–8.
13. Mato-Gondelle T, et al. Ultrasonographic findings in the vitreous of patients with age-related macular degeneration treated with intravitreal anti-vascular endothelial growth factor injections. Retina 2018;38(10):1962–7.

14. Zakov ZN, Berlin LA, Gutman FA. Ultrasonographic mapping of vitreoretinal abnormalities. Am J Ophthalmol. 1983;96(5):622–31.
15. Mamou J, et al. Ultrasound-based quantification of vitreous floaters correlates with contrast sensitivity and quality of life. Invest Ophthalmol. Visual Sci. 2015;56(3):1611–7.
16. Han S-S, et al. The use of contrast-enhanced color Doppler ultrasound in the differentiation of retinal detachment from vitreous membrane. Korean J Radiol. 2001;2(4):197.
17. Coleman DJ, et al. Explaining the current role of high-frequency ultrasound in ophthalmic diagnosis. Expert Rev Ophthalmol. 2006;1(1):63–76.
18. Dawood Z, Mirza SA, Qadeer A. Role of B-Scan ultrasonography for posterior segment lesions. JLUMHS 2008.
19. Palma J, Schott E. Acute, simultaneous, bilateral rhegmatogenous retinal detachment diagnosed with bedside emergency ultrasound. Am J Emerg Med. 2013;31(2):466-e3.
20. Agarwal A, et al. Characterization of retinal structure and diagnosis of peripheral acquired retinoschisis using high-resolution ultrasound B-scan. Graefe's Arch Clin Exp Ophthalmol. 2016;254(1):69–75.
21. Coleman DJ, Jack RL. B-scan ultrasonography in diagnosis and management of retinal detachments. Arch Ophthalmol. 1973;90(1):29–34.
22. Attia S, et al. Clinical and multimodal imaging characteristics of acute Vogt–Koyanagi–Harada disease unassociated with clinically evident exudative retinal detachment. International Ophthalmology 2016;36(1):37–44.
23. Karatas M, Ramirez JA, Ophir A. Diabetic vitreopapillary traction and macular oedema. Eye 2005;19:676–82.
24. Han DP, Lewandowski M, Mieler WF. Echographic diagnosis of anterior hyaloidal fibrovascular proliferation. Arch Ophthalmol. 1991;109(6):842–6.
25. Green W, Rao PK, Harocopos GJ. Extramedullary relapse of acute myelogenous leukemia presenting as a large serous retinal detachment. Ocular Oncol Pathol. 2017;3(2):95–100.
26. Mema V, Qafa N. Ocular complications of marfan syndrome. Report of two cases. Hippokratia 2010;14(1):45.
27. Johnson MW. Posterior vitreous detachment: evolution and complications of its early stages. Am J Ophthalmol. 2010;149(3):371–82.
28. van de Put MAJ, et al. Postoperative recovery of visual function after macula-off rhegmatogenous retinal detachment. PloS One 2014;9(6):e99787.
29. Kumar A, Sharma N, Singh R. Prone position ultrasonography in silicone filled eyes. Acta Ophthalmol Scand. 1998;76(4):496–8.
30. Pierro L, et al. Reliability of standardized echography before vitreoretinal surgery for proliferative diabetic retinopathy. Ophthalmologica 1998;212(Suppl. 1):91–2.
31. Jacobsen B, et al. Retrospective review of ocular point-of-care ultrasound for detection of retinal detachment. W J Emerg Med. 2016;17(2):196.
32. Zhang J, Zhu X-H, Tang L-S. Rhegmatogenous retinal detachment associated with massive spontaneous suprachoroidal hemorrhage and prognosis of pars plana vitrectomy. Int J Ophthalmol. 2014;7(5):850.
33. Dessì G, et al. Role of B-scan ocular ultrasound as an adjuvant for the clinical assessment of eyeball diseases: a pictorial essay. J Ultrasound 2015;18(3):265–77.
34. Zvornicanin J, et al. Significance of ultrasonography in evaluation of vitreo-retinal pathologies. Med Arch. 2012;66(5):318.
35. Abdolrahimzadeh S, et al. Spectral domain optical coherence tomography and B-scan ultrasonography in the evaluation of retinal tears in acute, incomplete posterior vitreous detachment. BMC Ophthalmol. 2016;16(1):1–9.
36. Blumenkranz MS, Byrne SF. Standardized echography (ultrasonography) for the detection and characterization of retinal detachment. Ophthalmology 1982;89(7):821–31.
37. Botwin A, Engel A, Wasyliw C. The use of ocular ultrasound to diagnose retinal detachment: a case demonstrating the sonographic findings. Emerg Radiol. 2018;25(4):445–7.

38. Okuda Y, et al. Two cases of rhegmatogenous retinal detachment associated with asteroid hyalosis. Case Rep Ophthalmol. 2018;9(1):49–54.
39. Ochi R, et al. Case of asteroid hyalosis that developed severely reduced vision after cataract surgery. BMC Ophthalmol. 2017;17(1):1–4.
40. Fuller DG, Laqua H, Machemer R. Ultrasonographic diagnosis of massive periretinal proliferation in eyes with opaque media (triangular retinal detachment). Am J Ophthalmol. 1977;83(4):460–4.
41. Shinar Z, Chan L, Orlinsky M. Use of ocular ultrasound for the evaluation of retinal detachment. J Emerg Med. 2011;40(1):53–7.
42. Stirpe M, Heimann K. Vitreous changes and retinal detachment in highly myopic eyes. Eur J Ophthalmol. 1996;6(1):50–8.
43. Maus M, Katz LJ. Choroidal detachment, flat anterior chamber, and hypotony as complications of neodymium: YAG laser cyclophotocoaguiation. Ophthalmology 1990;97 (1):69–72.
44. Vela MA, Campbell DG. Hypotony and ciliochoroidal detachment following pharmacologic aqueous suppressant therapy in previously filtered patients. Ophthalmology 1985;92(1):50–7.
45. Oksala A. Observations on choroidal detachment by means of ultrasound. Acta Ophthalmol. 1958;36(4):651–7.
46. Frost NA, Sparrow JM, Rosenthal AR. Posterior scleritis with retinal vasculitis and choroidal and retinal infarction. The Br J Ophthalmol. 1994;78(5):410.
47. Oksala A. The echogram in postoperative choroidal detachment. Acta Ophthalmol. 1962;40 (5):475–9.
48. Fledelius HC. Ultrasound in ophthalmology. Ultrasound Med Biol. 1997;23(3):365–75.
49. Jacobson DM. Intracranial hypertension and the syndrome of acquired hyperopia with choroidal folds. J Neuro-Ophthalmol: The Official J North Am Neuro-Ophthalmol Soc. 1995;15(3):178–85.
50. Byrne SF, Green RL. Ultrasound of the eye and orbit. 2nd ed. St. Louis: Mosby, Inc.; 2002.
51. Bhende M, et al. Atlas of ophthalmic ultrasound and ultrasound biomicroscopy. JP Medical Ltd. 2013.

Ocular Trauma

4

4.1 Anterior Segment

Ultrasound Biomicroscopy (UBM) provides valuable data about several structures in the anterior segment of the eye including cornea, angle of the anterior chamber, iris, ciliary body, lens and its zonules. It shows disruption of the normal appearance of intraocular structures such as iridodialysis, angle recession, cyclodialysis, Zonular rupture, and epithelial ingrowth, irrespective of the opaque media [21, 23]. It can also provide evidence for treatment. The surgical planning of anterior segment reconstruction depends on the data collected from UBM

4.1.1 Angle Recession

Angle recession is a tear into the ciliary body commonly caused by blunt trauma to the eye. On examination of pathological specimens, the tear is into the ciliary body itself, and does not produce disinsertion of the ciliary body from the scleral spur. The superficial aspect of the tear can have a high reflectivity most likely representing secondary condensation of the ciliary body tissue on this surface [1] (Fig. 4.1).

4.1.2 Cyclodialysis

Cyclodialysis refers to the disinsertion of the ciliary body from the scleral spur. Formation of cyclodialysis clefts allows a direct communication between the anterior chamber and the suprachoroidal space [2]. Clinically the pupil is irregular, being displaced toward the site of the cyclodialysis [25, 26] (Fig. 4.2).

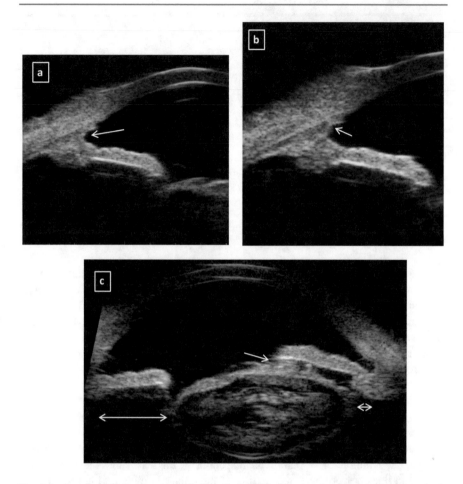

Fig. 4.1 A case of angle recession. **a** longitudinal UBM scan showing a tear in the ciliary body (white arrow). **b** The inner surface of a ciliary body tear shows a high reflectivity (white arrow), most likely representing condensation of ciliary body tissue, where the ciliary body remains attached at the scleral spur. **c** Axial UBM scan of the same patient showing subluaxated cataractous lens shifted to the opposite side (short double arrow) denoting zonular rupture at that side (long double arrow) with the lens pushed anteriorly, as well as evidence of anterior capsule dehiscence with lens matter protrusion (white arrow)

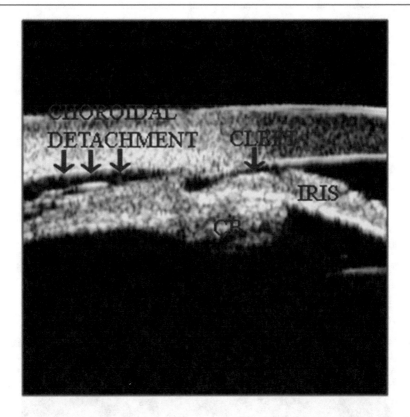

Fig. 4.2 Ultrasound biomicroscopy (UBM) is probably the most sensitive technique for detecting an active cyclodialysis cleft. CB ciliary body (From Gonzalez Martin-Moro et al. Int Ophthalmol (2017) 37:441–457) [25]

4.1.3 Iridodialysis

Traumatic iridodialysis the iris tends to tear at its thinnest area near the root resulting in a wide-angle appearance, which differs from the ultrasound biomicroscopic appearance of an iridectomy, where the iridectomy is more medial in location and shows a small residual portion of the iris root remaining peripherally [1, 12] (Figs. 4.3, 4.4, 4.5 and 4.6).

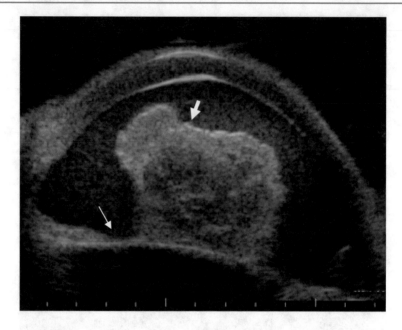

Fig. 4.3 UBM scan of hyphemia with clotted blood (thick arrow) attached to the anterior capsule (thin arrow) which obscure the details of the anterior chamber on clinical examintion

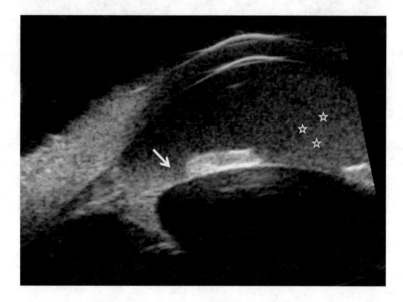

Fig. 4.4 Longitudinal UBM scan showing hyphemia, appears as echoes filling the anterior chamber (stars), with the iridodialysis (white arrow) detected by the UBM

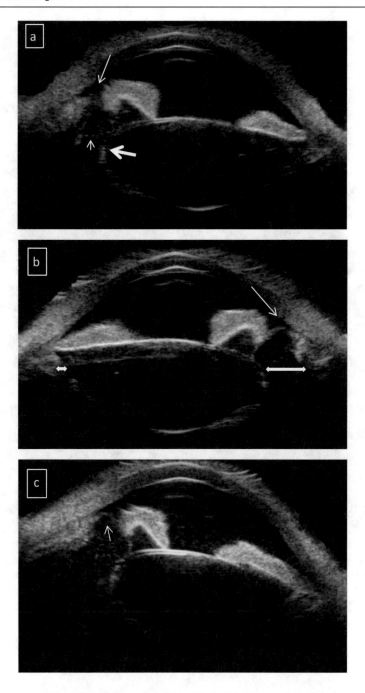

Fig. 4.5 A case of iridodialysis: **a** showing iridodialysis (thin arrow) with zonular rupture (short arrow), with spherical edge of the lens (thick arrow) in the region of zonular rupture. **b** and **c** UBM scan above the iridodialysis with vitreous herniating in the anterior chamber (white arrow), and demonstrating shifting of the lens to the opposite side (double arrows in **b** showing the distance between the cilliary body and the lens equater in opposite sides)

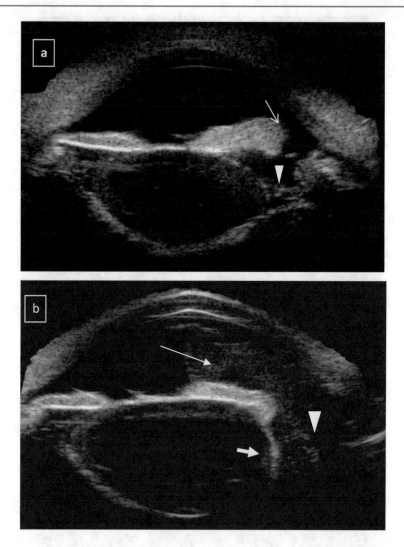

Fig. 4.6 a UBM scan above the edge of iridodialysis (white arrow) showing the intact zonules (triangle) underneath. **b** UBM Scan above the iridodialysis with vitreous herniating in the anterior chamber (thin arrow) as well as zonular rupture (triangle) with spherical contour (thick arrow) of the lens equator in the region of missed zonules

4.1.4 Traumatic Lens and IOL Disorders

UBM is an effective method for evaluating traumatic lens disorders including change in zonular tension or loss of zonules. The normal lens equator changes to a rounded shape, when there is loss or laxity of the zonules in that quadrant [3, 8, 9]. UBM can also help identifying anterior or posterior capsular dehiscence [7, 18] (Figs. 4.7, 4.8, 4.9 and 4.10).

UBM is also a useful tool in detecting the tilt, decentration of the IOL and the exact location of haptics in relation to the normal anatomic landmarks [11] (Figs. 4.11, 4.12 and 4.13).

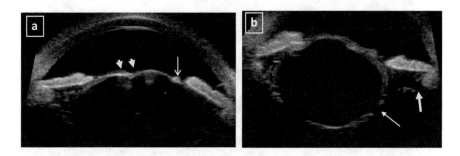

Fig. 4.7 A case of penetrating trauma. **a** Axial UBM scan showing irregular opened anterior capsule (short arrows) with lens matter protrusion (thin arrow). **b** Spherical lens equator due to zonular rupture (thick arrow) with the lens pushed anteriorly showing evidence of posterior capsule tear (thin arrow)

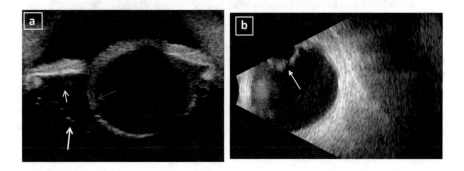

Fig. 4.8 The same patient. **a** Exposing the zonular rupture (thin arrow) with shifting of the lens to the opposite quadrant and spherical lens equator (red arrow) in the region of missed zonules, with vitreous strands underneath (thick arrow), **b** longitudinal B-scan showing irregular posterior capsule (denoting the posterior capsule dehiscence) (white arrow)

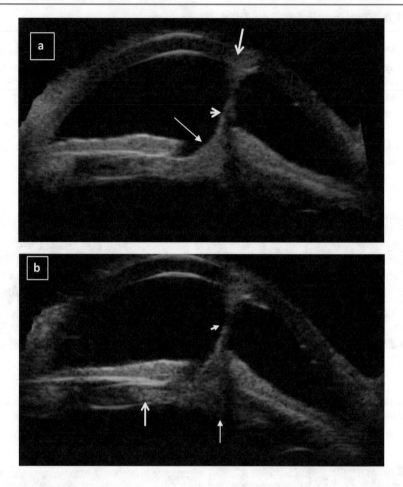

Fig. 4.9 Penetrating wound with a needle. **a** Corneal wound (thick arrow) showing track of entrance of the needle (short arrow in **a** and **b**) connected to the ruptured anterior lens capsule (thin arrow) (denoting the depth of penetration), **b** Ruptured posterior lens capsule (thin arrow), with partially absorbed lens (thick arrow)

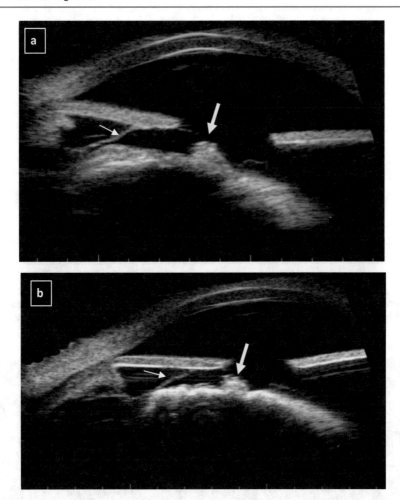

Fig. 4.10 A case of penetrating trauma **a** subluxated lens with irregular ruptured anterior lens capsule with lens matter protrusion (thick arrows in **a** and **b**), **b** revealing the vitreous strand passing between the iris and the subluxated lens (thin arrow)

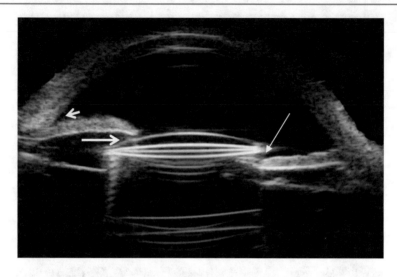

Fig. 4.11 A case of blunt trauma after Cataract surgery, An axial UBM scan showing pupillary capture IOL, with one edge of the IOL above the pupillary edge (thin arrow) and the opposite IOL edge below the iris (thick arrow), with iris bombe causing narrowing of the angle (short arrow)

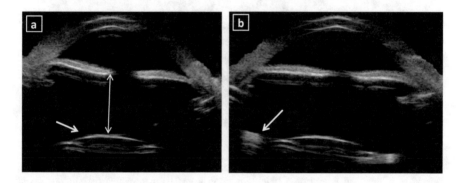

Fig. 4.12 **a** A Dislocated IOL (thick arrow) in the anterior vitreous cavity (double arrow showing distance between the iris and the dislocated IOL), **b** An axial UBM scan showing the haptic of the IOL (white arrow)

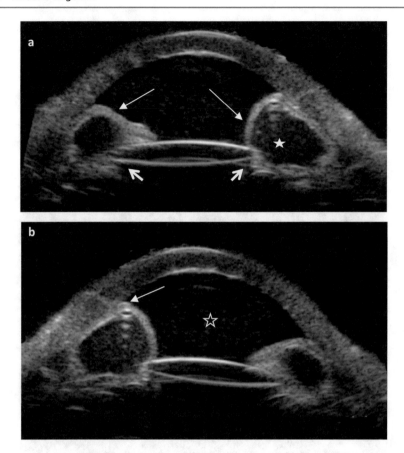

Fig. 4.13 Axial UBM scans **a** showing 2 large iris cysts (white arrows) at nasal and temporal side pushing the iris forward causing iridocorneal adhesion obliterating the angle, with multiple echoes filling the iris cyst (stars), subluxated IOL with the IOL edges embedded in the iris tissue (short arrows), b note the suture passing from the cornea into the iris tissue (white arrow) and the echoes filling the anterior chamber (inflammatory cells) (star)

4.1.5 Foreign Bodies (F.B)

UBM helps in detection and accurate localization of anterior chamber foreign bodies till the pars plana and peripheral retina [10]. It detects small, nonmetallic and anteriorly located foreign bodies which can be missed by CT scan (Figs. 4.14, 4.15, 4.16 and 4.17).

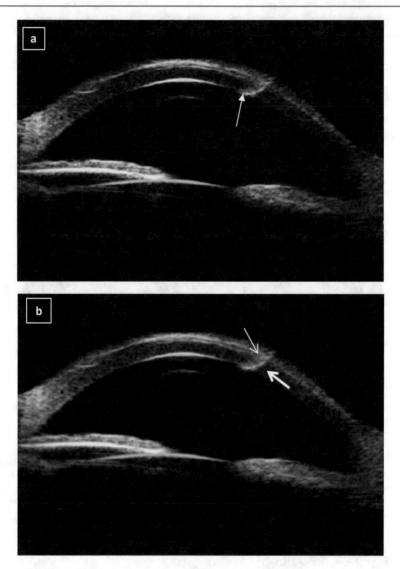

Fig. 4.14 Intracorneal foreign body: **a** Tiny metallic foreign body embedded in the posterior cornea (white arrow), **b** showing the track of entrance of the foreign body (thick arrow) which caused corneal oedema (thin arrow) obscuring visualization of the foreign body by clinical examination

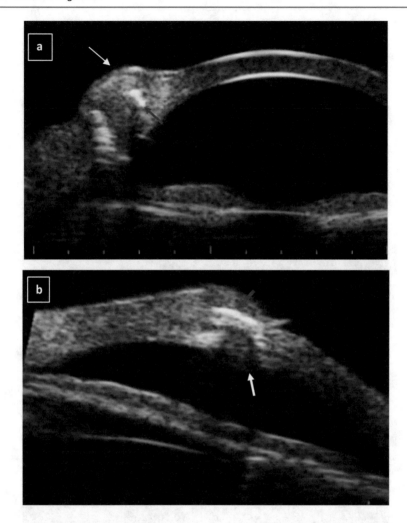

Fig. 4.15 **a** A patient with a granuloma (white arrow) at the limbus where an impacted foreign body (red arrows) discovered by UBM, **b** Transverse UBM scan of the foreign body revealing more about its dimensions, with evidence of shadowing of the foreign body underneath (white arrow)

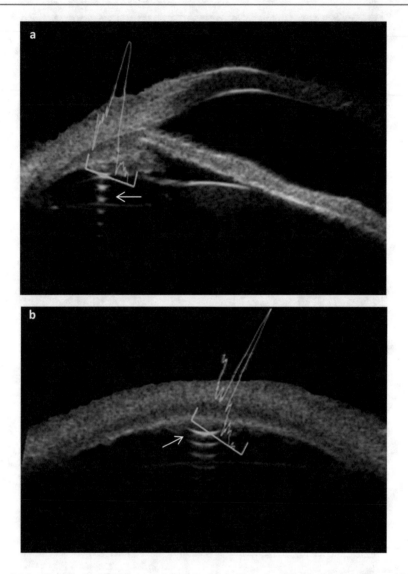

Fig. 4.16 **a** Longitudinal UBM scan of glass foreign body in the ciliary body producing multiple signals behind it (white arrow), **b** Transverse UBM scan exposing the foreign body (white arrow) for prober localization and measurment, with high reflectivity in superimposed A-scan

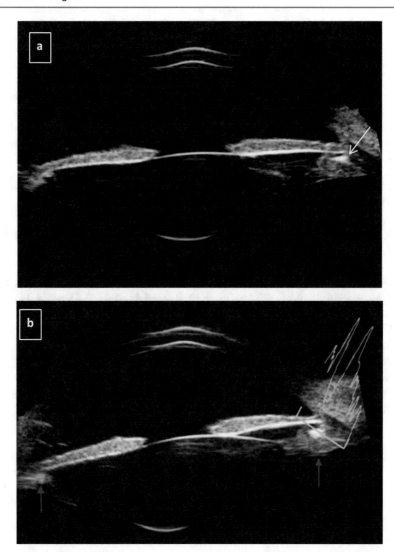

Fig. 4.17 a Axial UBM scan showing foreign body (white arrow) embedded in the ciliary body more evident with decreasing the gain **b** the foreign body with high reflictivity in the superimposed A-scan, note the swelling of the cilliary body compared to the cilliary body in the opposite side (red arrows)

4.2   Posterior Segment

Ocular trauma can cause tissue damage, varying in severity from minor injuries to medical emergencies. There are different forms of trauma, including penetrating, blunt or surgical traumas, which can produce tissue damage in varying degrees, temporarily or permanently compromising visual function.

B-scan ultrasonography has been shown to yield valuable diagnostic and prognostic information to define the nature of the pathology and guide management [4, 5, 6, 13, 19]. It is used in ocular trauma to assess:

1. Internal ocular damage/anatomy following trauma in eyes with opaque media
2. Traumatic cataract and dislocated lens/IOL [14, 15] (Figs. 4.18, 4.19, 4.20, 4.21, 4.22 and 4.23).
3. Vitreous hemorrhage and hemorrhagic track through the vitreous (Figs. 4.27, 4.28, 4.29 and 4.30)
4. Traumatic endophthalmitis (Fig. 4.58)
5. Detection and localization of intraocular foreign bodies [22] (Figs. 4.31, 4.32, 4.33, 4.34, 4.35, 4.36, 4.37, 4.38, 4.39, 4.40, 4.41, 4.42, 4.43 and 4.44).
6. Retinal tears and detachments (Figs. 4.24, 4.25 and 4.26).
7. Differentiation between serous and hemorrhagic choroidal detachments and follow-up for clot lysis (Figs. 4.51, 4.52, 4.53 and 4.54).
8. Avulsion of optic disc (Fig. 4.57).
9. Scleral rupture [16] (Figs. 4.45, 4.46)
10. Posterior exit wounds with associated incarceration of intraocular contents [17, 20] (Figs. 4.47, 4.48, 4.49, 4.50, 4.55 and 4.56).

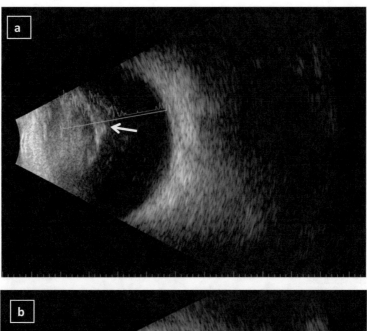

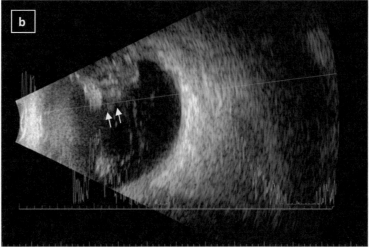

Fig. 4.18 Posterior capsular dehiscence due to penetrating trauma. **a** Axial B-scan showing irregular posterior capsule (white arrow). **b** Longitudinal B-scan showing opened posterior capsule with lens matter protrusion (white arrows). **c** the same patient with lens fragment (white arrow) in the vitreous cavity of high reflectivity in the superimposed A-scan

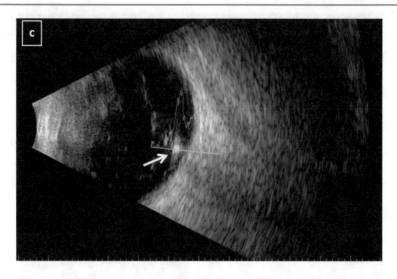

Fig. 4.18 (continued)

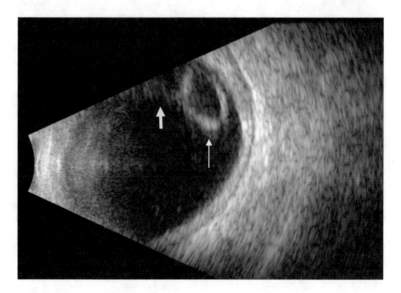

Fig. 4.19 Dislocated lens in the vitreous cavity (thin arrow) attached to it vitreous track (thick arrow)

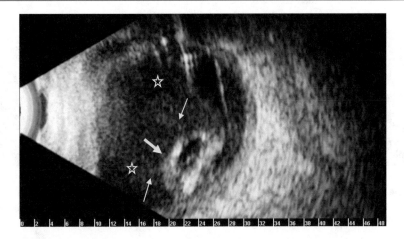

Fig. 4.20 Blunt trauma causing dislocated cataractous lens, oval in shape (thick arrow), with dense vitreous hemorrhage (stars) and vitreous membranes attached to the lens (thin arrows)

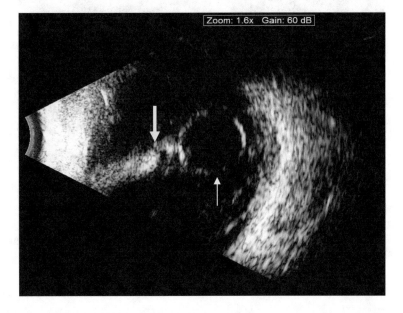

Fig. 4.21 Dislocated clear lens, spherical in shape (thin arrow) with vitreous track attached to it (white thick arrow)

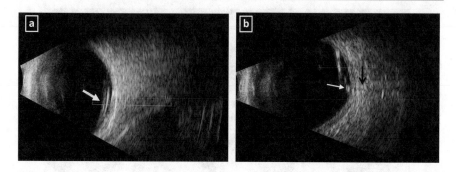

Fig. 4.22 **a** Dislocated IOL showing high reflective surface (white arrow) with high amplitude in superimposed A-scan. **b** showing the haptic (white arrow) of the dislocated IOL causing mild shadowing to the orbital tissue posteriorly (black arrow)

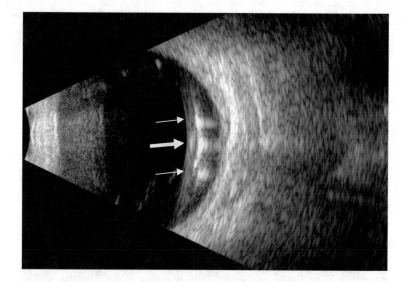

Fig. 4.23 Dislocated Iris claw IOL (white arrow) with high reflective surface, showing the haptics (thin arrows)

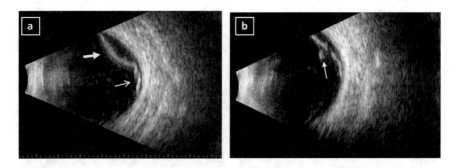

Fig. 4.24 **a** Transverse scan showing mild vitreous haemorrhage after blunt trauma with retinal detachment (thick arrow), evidence of retinal tear (white arrow), **b** longitudnal scan showing the retinal tear with residual attachment of the posterior hyaloid to the tear (white arrow)

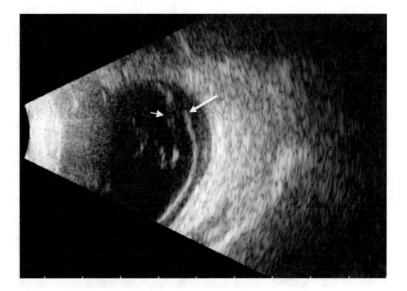

Fig. 4.25 Large peripheral retinal tear (white long arrow) in the inferonasal quadrant anteriorly after penetrating trauma, with attachment of a fine hemorrhagic track to one edge of the tear (short arrow)

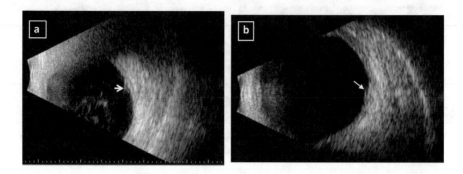

Fig. 4.26 a Retinal tear in the superior quadrant after blunt trauma, **b** longitudnal scan showing the retinal flap (white arrow)

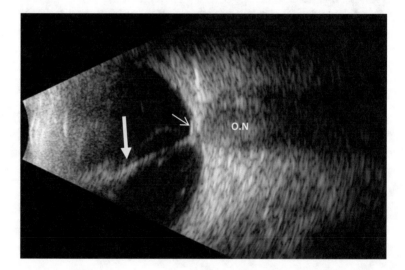

Fig. 4.27 Penetrating trauma with vitreous track (thick arrow) extending from the anterior segment to the retina round the optic nerve (O.N) causing shallow detachment (thin arrow)

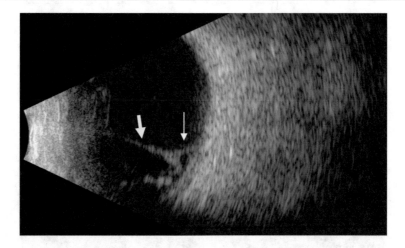

Fig. 4.28 Another patient with penetrating trauma showing vitreous track (white arrow) extending from the anterior segment to the retina causing focal traction retinal detachment (thin arrow) in the inferior quadrant

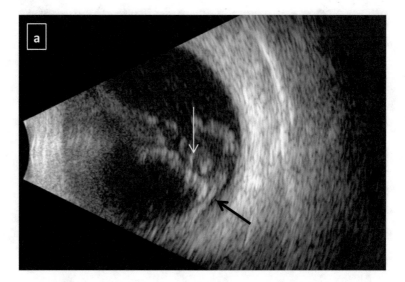

Fig. 4.29 a Transverse scan showing vitreous track (white arrow) extending from anterior segment to be attached to a shallow detached retina (black arrow), **b**: longitudinal scan showing the extension of the detached retina (arrow)

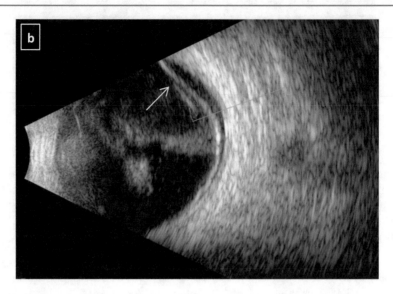

Fig. 4.29 (continued)

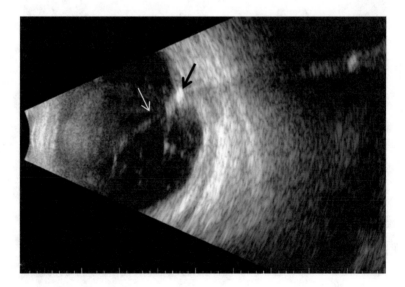

Fig. 4.30 Haemorrhagic track (white arrow) leading to a metallic foreign body (black arrow) impacted in the retina

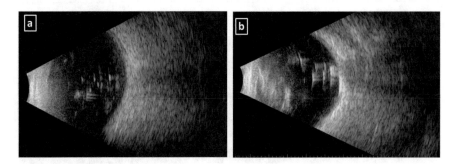

Fig. 4.31 Repaired rupture globe after a car accident with broken glasses **a** showing multiple echoes in the vitreous cavity of low to moderate echogenicity, **b** Different probe positions were applied to allow the sound beam to streak the flat surface of the glasses producing the significant multiple signals behind

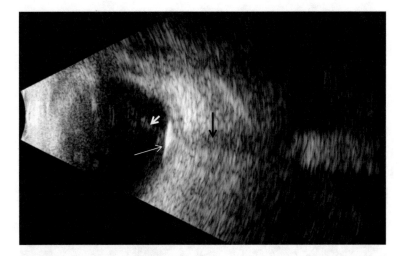

Fig. 4.32 Intraocular foreign body laying on the retina (thin arrow) causing shadowing to the orbital tissue posteriorly (black arrow), note the vitreous track (short arrow)

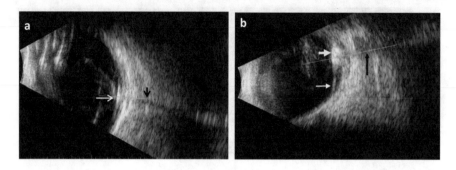

Fig. 4.33 **a** Transverse scan showing metal foreign body (white arrow) of high echogenicity causing shadowing to the orbital tissue posteriorly (black arrow), **b** longitudinal scan leading to more exposure of the foreign body for proper localization and accurate measurement (thick arrow) impacted in the retina causing retinal detachment (thin arrow), Note the shadowing to the orbital tissue (black arrow)

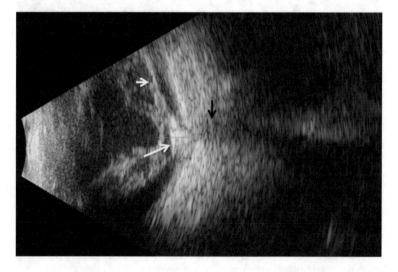

Fig. 4.34 Intraocular foreign body impacted in the retina (long arrow) with retinal detachment at its side (short arrow), causing shadowing to the orbital tissue behind it (black arrow)

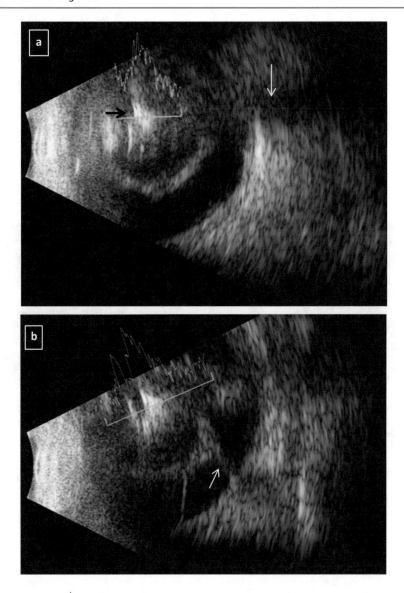

Fig. 4.35 **a** longstanding nail foreign body (black arrow) in the anterior vitreous cavity of high echogenicity and high amplitude on A-scan, causing shadowing to the orbital tissues posteriorly (white arrow), **b** exposing the longstanding total retinal detachment with closed funnel posteriorly (arrow)

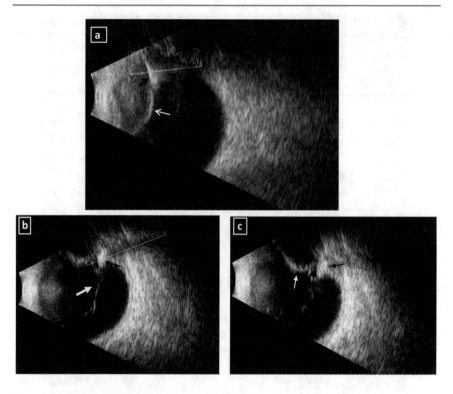

Fig. 4.36 a Paraxial scan showing a foreign body (black arrow) next to the lens (white arrow),
b and **c** Longitudinal scan exposing the anteriorly located metallic foreign body (black arrow), note
the vitreous track (arrow in **b**) and the opaque lens (arrow in **c**)

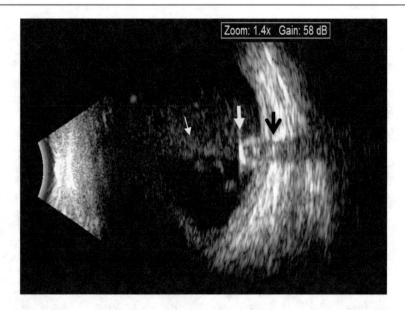

Fig. 4.37 Metallic foreign body (thick arrow) in the vitreous cavity causing shadowing to the orbital tissue (black arrow), with haemorrhagic track (thin arrow), note the low gain used for accurate identification of the foreign body

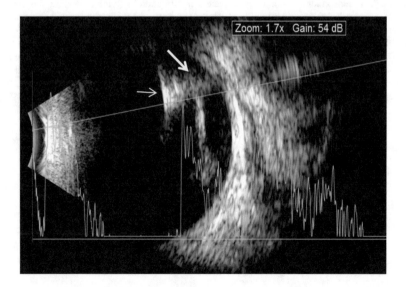

Fig. 4.38 Spherical foreign body (BBs) (thin arrow) in the vitreous cavity with characteristic chain of multiple signals decreasing in amplitude known as comet tail artifacts (thick arrow), which is a specific echographic signal for spherical metallic F.Bs

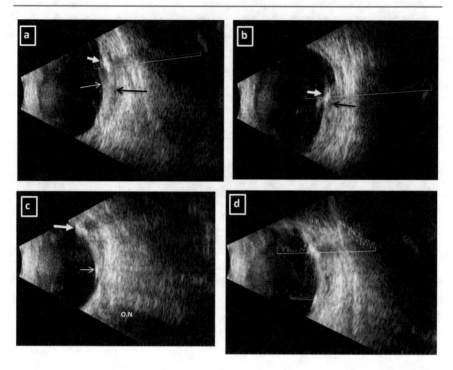

Fig. 4.39 a Intraocular foreign body impacted in the choroid (thick arrow) in the temporal quadrant anteriorly causing subretinal hemorrhage and choroidal thickening, which appear as one thick layer (thin white arrow), with mobile echoes between the retina and choroid in kinetic scan. As well as suprachoroidal hemorrhage seen as mobile echoes in the suprachoroidal space (black arrow), **b** Transverse scan with another foreign body (white arrow) impacted in the retina in temporal quadrant central with subretinal hemorrhage (black arrow) (**c** and **d**) Longitudinal scans showing the two intraocular foreign body: One foreign body temporal to the optic nerve (O.N) and another one in temporal quadrant anteriorly (thick arrow) with their A-scan of high reflectivity (**d**)

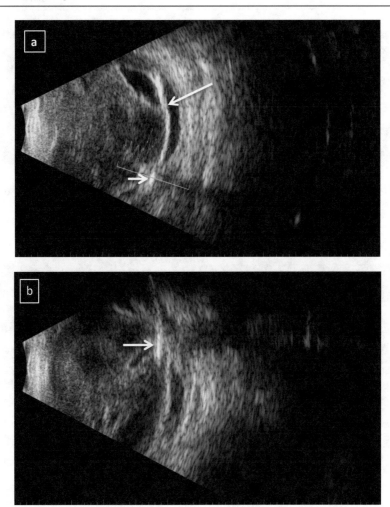

Fig. 4.40 **a** Transverse scan showing retinal detachment (long arrow) and small intraocular foreign body (short arrow), **b** longitudinal scan for more exposure of the foreign body (white arrow) and accurate estimation of its diminutions

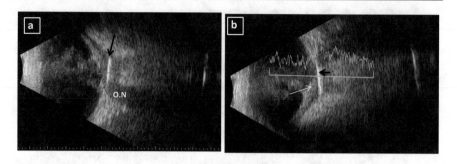

Fig. 4.41 a Longitudnal scan of I.O.F.B (black arrow) inferotemporal to the optic nerve (O.N).
b Transverse scan showing the F.B (black arrow) impacted in the choroid (white arrow), Note the
high reflectivity of the F.B in A-scan

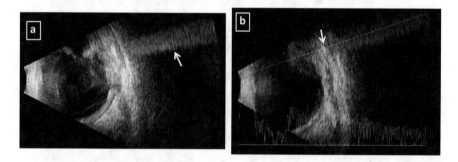

Fig. 4.42 a An artifacts seen posteriorly (white arrow) denoting the presence of a F.B, **b** for
revealing the retrobulbar F.B (white arrow) the patient was examined at low gain setting, as F.Bs
will not disappear even by lowering the gain, note the high reflectivity of the F.B in A-scan

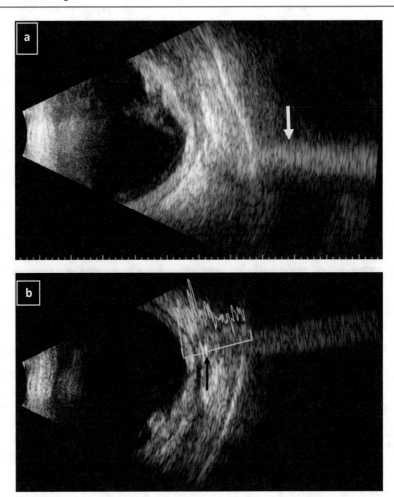

Fig. 4.43 a Retrobulbar F.B recognized by the produced artifacts (white arrow) where the F.B. can't be easily differentiated from the high echogenicity of the surrounding orbital tissues, **b** By lowering the gain setting the F.B can be differentiated from the surrounding tissue (black arrow), Note its high amplitude in A-scan

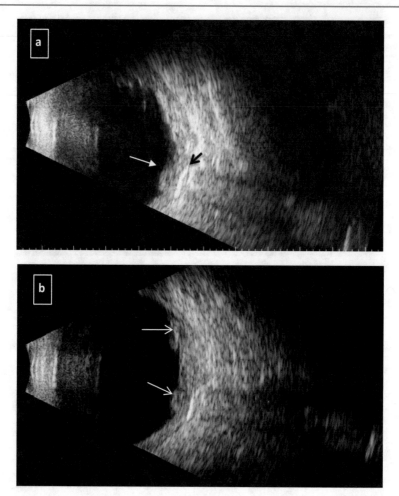

Fig. 4.44 **a** I.O.F.B (black arrow) impacted in the sclera with irregular surface of the retina and choroid around it (white arrow), **b** lowering the gain setting for more exposure of the F.B and revealing the extent of the affected retina and choroid (white arrows)

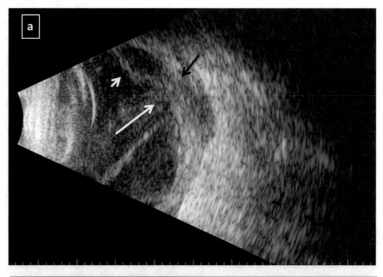

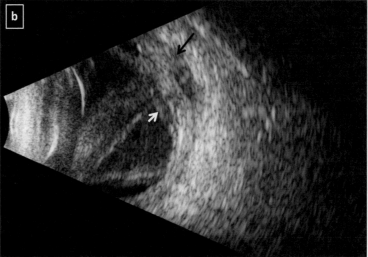

Fig. 4.45 a Longitudinal scan showing peripheral posterior scleral rupture (black arrows) following perforating ocular injury, with vitreous track incarcerated in the posterior rupture (long arrow) and retinal incarceration causing detachment around the posterior perforation (short arrows) (**a** and **b**)

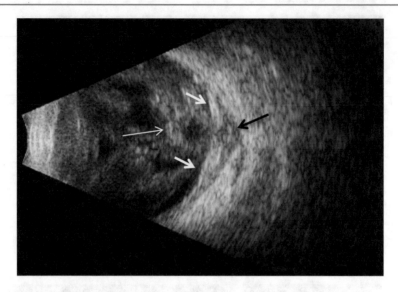

Fig. 4.46 Transverse scan of a patient with posterior scleral rupture (black arrow), with irregular thickening of the retina and choroid (short arrows) around the scleral rupture note the vitreous track incarceration (white long arrow)

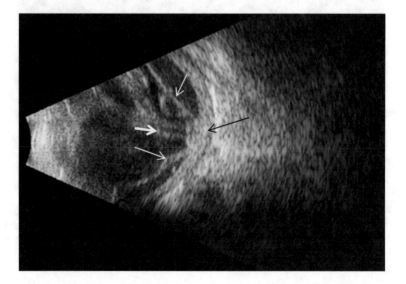

Fig. 4.47 Transverse scan of another patient revealing choroidal rupture with choroidal hematoma (black arrow), with vitreous track (white thick arrow) and retinal incarceration in the posterior rupture, causing retinal detachment around the rupture (white thin arrows)

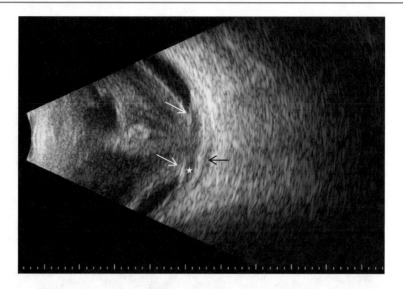

Fig. 4.48 Transverse scan of another patient with perforating trauma with choroidal irregularity (suggestive of choroidal rupture) with hemorrhage in suprachoroidal space (black arrow), and elevated retina (white arrows) by subretinal haemorrhage (star), and vitreous track incarceration (red arrow)

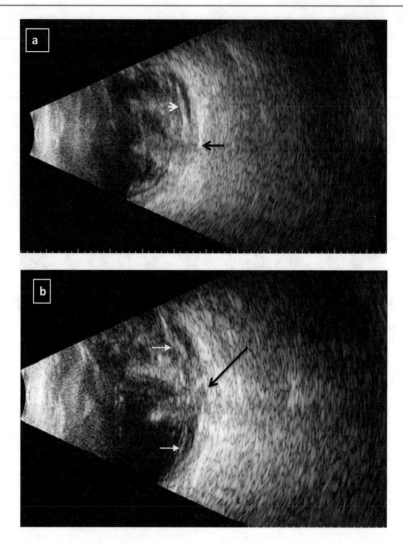

Fig. 4.49 a Transverse scan and **b** longitudinal scan of perforating trauma showing an exist wound (black arrows) with vitreous track and retina incarcerated, with retinal detachment (white arrows) around it extending anteriorly

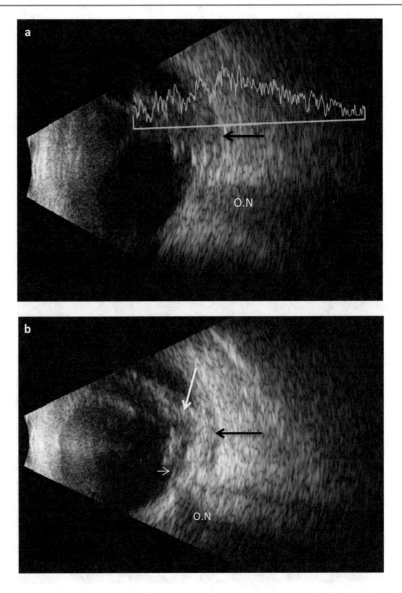

Fig. 4.50 a Posterior perforation (black arrows) inferotemporal to the optic disc (O.N) involving the macular area, with irregular thickening of the choroid underneath and with irregular reflectivity on A-scan **b** Longitudinal scan showing the vitreous track incarceration (white arrow) and retina from the optic disc to the posterior rupture elevated by subretinal hemorrhage (white short arrow)

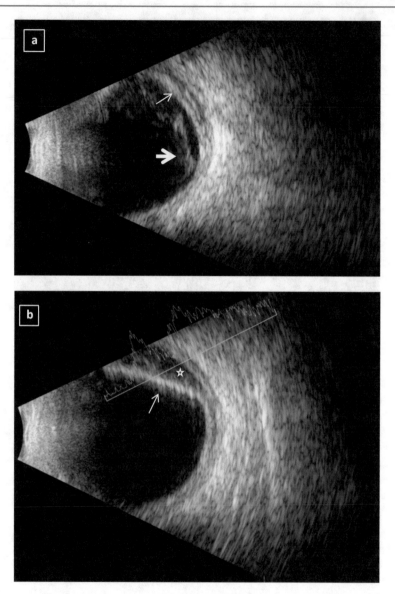

Fig. 4.51 A case of repired rupture globe after penetrating trauma **a** longitudinal scan of one quadrant with shallow choroidal separation (thin arrow), and vitreous hemorrhage (white thick arrow), **b** longitudinal scan of another quadrant with ciliochoroidal detachment (white arrow) and suprachoroidal hemorrhage (star)

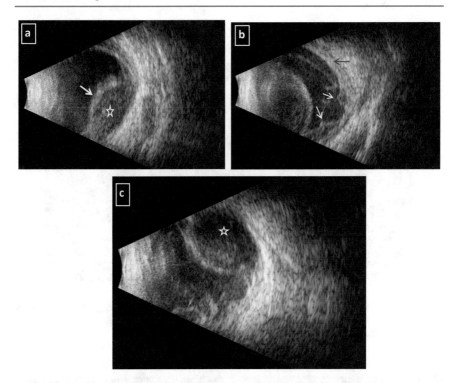

Fig. 4.52 Hemorrhagic choroidal detachment in the nasal and inferior quadrant after penetrating injury, **a** Transverse scan of the nasal quadrant showing choroidal detachment (white arrow) with suprachoroidal hemorrhage (star), **b** Transverse scan showing the temporal quadrant with multiple focal tractional retinal detachment (white arrows) and choroidal thickening (red arrow), **c** longitudinal scan of the nasal quadrant exposing the anterior end of the choroidal detachment with hemorrhage filling the suprachoroidal space (star)

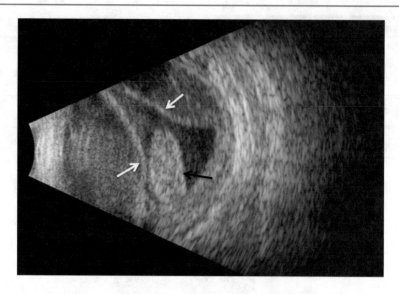

Fig. 4.53 Another case of haemorrhagic choroidal detachment showing organized hemorrhage (black arrow) in the vitreous cavity, with oppositional choroidal detachment (white arrows), and suprachoroidal hemorrhage

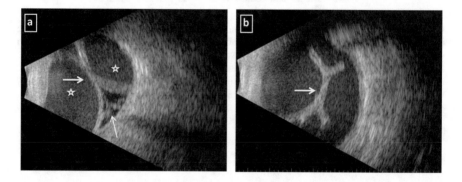

Fig. 4.54 Another case of traumatic hemorrhagic choroidal detachment Kissing choroid with **a** longitudinal scan showing adherent (kissing) choroid (white arrow) with suprachoroidal hemorrhage (stars), and evidence of shallow retinal detachment at posterior edge of choroidal detachment (white thin arrow) **b** Transverse scan of the kissing choroid (white arrow)

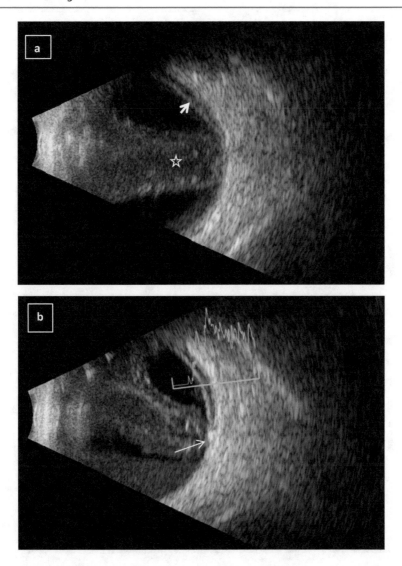

Fig. 4.55 Penetrating needle injury during retrobulbar anesthesia **a** transverse scan showing vitreous hemorrhage (star) with vitreous incarceration and retinal detachment (white arrow), **b** A longitudinal scan for more exposure of the site of penetration (white arrow) and the extend of retinal detachment

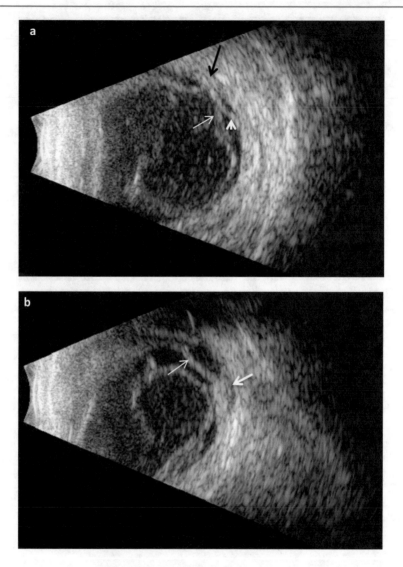

Fig. 4.56 Penetrating needle injury during retrobulbar anesthesia (black arrow) **a** Transverse scan showing vitreous incarceration (white thin arrow) and localized retinal detachment around the site of posterior needle penetration (white short arrow). **b** A longitudinal scan with more exposure of the site of posterior penetration which caused a localized choroidal thickening (thick arrow) (suggestive of choroidal hematoma) with localized choroidal detachment (thin arrow)

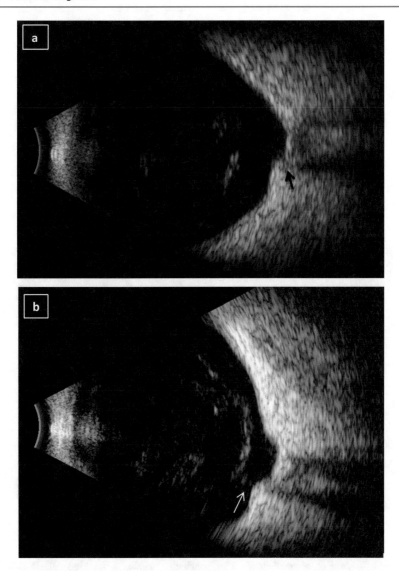

Fig. 4.57 Acute avulsion of optic nerve after severe blunt trauma **a** Axial scan showing irregular appearance of the optic nerve head (due to retraction of the oedematous optic nerve into its sheath), with scleral rupture at the edge of the optic disc (black arrow), **b** longitudinal scan showing hemorrhagic track emanating from the edge of the optic disc

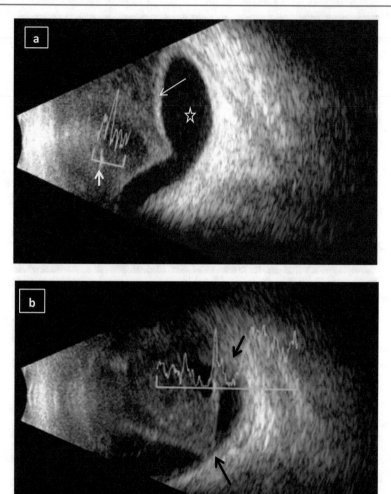

Fig. 4.58 A case of endophthalmitis after penetrating trauma. **a** An intraocular F.B in the retrolental space (white short arrow) surrounded with echoes of moderate amplitude in the vitreous cavity, with thickened posterior hyaloid (white thin arrow) and echoes of low echogenicity in the subhyaloid space (star) denoting active inflammtion **b** longitudnal scan showing multiple points of posterior hyaloid attachment to the retina (black arrows), **c** longitudnal scan showing organized vitreous membranes attached to the retina anteriorly (black arrow), note the opaque lens (white thin arrow)

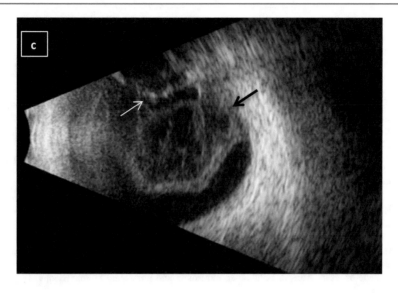

Fig. 4.58 (continued)

References

1. Pavlin CJ, Stuart Foster F. Ultrasound biomicroscopy of the eye. Springer Science & Business Media; 2012.
2. Özdal MPÇ, Mansour M, Deschenes J. Ultrasound biomicroscopic evaluation of the traumatized eyes. Eye. 2003;17(4):467–72.
3. Pavlin CJ, Buys YM, Pathmanathan T. Imaging zonular abnormalities using ultrasound biomicroscopy. Arch Ophthalmol. 1998;116(7):854–7.
4. lmendárez JE, et al. Ultrasound findings in ocular trauma. Archivos de la Sociedad Española de Oftalmol (English Edition). 2015;90(12):572–7.
5. McNicholas MM, et al. Ocular trauma: evaluation with US. Radiology. 1995;195(2):423–7.
6. Rubsamen PE, et al. Diagnostic ultrasound and pars plana vitrectomy in penetrating ocular trauma. Ophthalmology. 1994;101(5):809–14.
7. Tabatabaei A, et al. Evaluation of posterior lens capsule by 20-MHz ultrasound probe in traumatic cataract. Am J Ophthalmol. 2012;153(1):51–4.
8. Dhar M, et al. Is UBM useful for zonular intergrity?. Kerala J Ophthalmol. 4(1):144.
9. Salehi-Had H, Turalba A. Management of traumatic crystalline lens subluxation and dislocation. Int Ophthalmol Clin. 2010;50(1):167–79.
10. Parija S, Behera P, Banerjee A, et al. Ultrasound biomicroscopy for ophthalmology–an overview. J Evid Based Med Healthc. 2017;4(59):3589–94. https://doi.org/10.18410/jebmh/2017/715.
11. Ceylan OM, et al. Ultrasound biomicroscopic findings of blunt eye traumas. Gülhane Tip Dergisi. 2011;53(1):31.
12. Romanazzi F, Morano A, Caccavale A. Diagnostic and therapeutic approach in a case of severe post-traumatic hyphema with subtotal iridodialysis. Case Rep Ophthalmol. 2017;8(3):496–502.
13. Blaivas M, Theodoro D, Sierzenski PR. A study of bedside ocular ultrasonography in the emergency department. Acad Emerg Med. 2002;9(8):791–9.

14. Frasure SE, Saul T, Lewiss RE. Bedside ultrasound diagnosis of vitreous hemorrhage and traumatic lens dislocation. Am J Emerg Med. 2013;31(6):1002-e1.
15. Haghighi SHO, et al. Diagnostic accuracy of ultrasound in detection of traumatic lens dislocation. Emergency. 2014;2(3):121.
16. Oksala A, Lehtinen A. Diagnostics of rupture of the sclera by means of ultrasound. Acta Ophthalmol. 1958;36(1):37–42.
17. Wadood AC, Dhillon B, Singh J. Inadvertent ocular perforation and intravitreal injection of an anesthetic agent during retrobulbar injection. J Cataract Refract Surg. 2002;28(3):562–5.
18. Kumawat D, et al. Posttraumatic isolated posterior capsule rupture with posterior dislocation of lens nucleus. JCRS Online Case Rep. 2017;5(3):49–51.
19. Kramer M, Hart Lois, Miller JW. Ultrasonography in the management of penetrating ocular trauma. 1995.
20. Schneider ME, et al. Ocular perforation from a retrobulbar injection. Am J Ophthalmol. 1988;106(1):35–40.
21. Heur M, Jeng BH. Anterior segment disorders. Ultrasound Clin. 2008;3(2):201–6.
22. Kükner AŞ, et al. Characteristics of pellet injuries to the orbit. Ophthalmologica. 2009;223 (6):390–5.
23. Elshafie M, et al. Ultrasonic evaluation of eyes with blunt trauma. J Egypt Ophthalmol Soc. 2018;111(1): 20–20.
24. Bhende M, et al. Atlas of ophthalmic ultrasound and ultrasound biomicroscopy. JP Medical Ltd.; 2013.
25. González-Martín-Moro J, et al. Cyclodialysis: an update. Int Ophthalmol. 2017;37(2):441–57.
26. Park M, Kondo T. Ultrasound biomicroscopic findings in a case of cyclodialysis. Ophthalmologica. 1998;212(3):194–7.

Congenital Anomalies and Pediatric Eye Diseases

5

5.1 Limbal Dermoid

Limbal dermoids are uncommon choristomatous corneal tumors. They are clinically present as round or oval, whitish or yellowish masses on the anterior surface of the eyeball. A study by Nevares et al. indicates that the majority (76%) of ocular dermoids occur at the inferotemporal with the other 22% reported to occur superotemporally [7].

Choriostomas may or may not be associated with systemic conditions and other syndromes, such as ring dermoid syndrome with conjunctival extension, preauricular tags, palpebral coloboma, Goldenhar's syndrome (preauricular fistulae, preauricular appendages, and epibulbar dermoids or lipodermoids), as well as the mandibulofacial dysostosis of Franceschetti syndrome. Goldenhar's syndrome has been expanded further to include vertebral anomalies and is now named Goldenhar-Gorlin syndrome [7].

Epibulbar dermoid are composed of inclusions of epidermal and sometimes mesodermal tissues. Histologically,these tumors are composed of collagenous connective tissue covered by stratified squamous epithelium. Dermal appendages such as hair follicles and sebaceous glands often extend into the underlying tissue [1].

Limbal dermoid grades

(A) *Grade I pediatric limbal dermoids:* with superficial corneal involvement, management is initially conservative.
(B) *Grade II pediatric limbal dermoids:* affecting the full thickness of the cornea with/without endothelial involvement.

R. Abbas, *Ophthalmic Ultrasonography and Ultrasound Biomicroscopy*,
https://doi.org/10.1007/978-3-030-76979-6_5

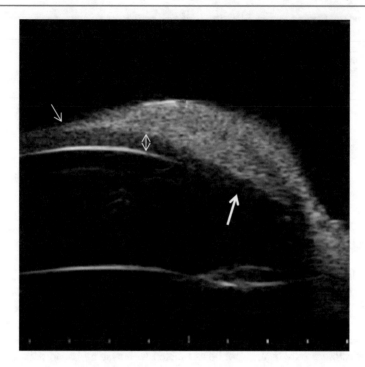

Fig. 5.1 Large Limbal dermoid reaching almost the center of the cornea (thin arrow)with infiltration of corneal stroma leaving 0.3 mm of cornea layers intact underneath(double arrow), with the high echogenicity of the lesion there is less visibility of the posterior corneal surface as it reaches the limbus due to sound attention

(C) *Grade III pediatric limbal dermoids*: involving the entire cornea and anterior chamber. A combination of excision, lamellar keratoplasty, and amniotic membrane and limbal stem cell transplantation are advocated [41].

Knowing the depth of the lesion is important in surgical planning. which may vary from simple shaving and conjunctival closure, to extreme cases of fashioning a customized corneal or scleral graft to replace the excised tissue [5, 30] (Figs. 5.1, 5.2, 5.3, 5.4, 5.5 and 5.6).

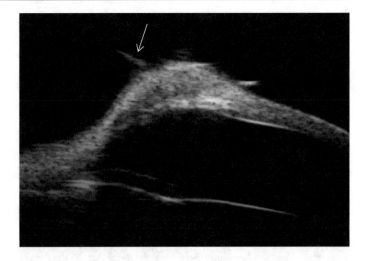

Fig. 5.2 Limbal dermoid infiltrating almost all the corneal layers sparing the endothelium, with evidence of protruding hair (white arrow)

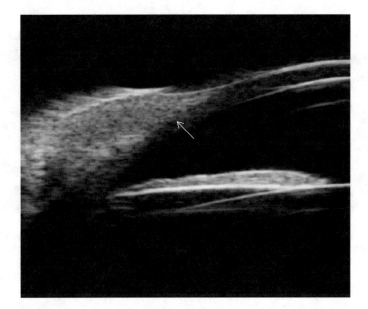

Fig. 5.3 Limbal dermoid of high echogenicity showing infiltration of the corneal stroma (arrow) with less visibility of the posterior cornea due to sound attenuation, with no evidence of anterior chamber infiltration

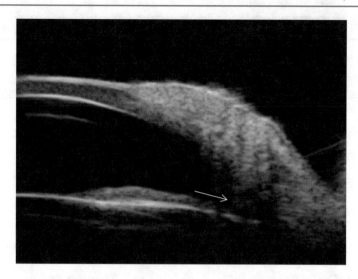

Fig. 5.4 Limbal dermoid infiltrating all corneal layer and entering the anterior chamber towards the angle causing sound attenuation to the anterior surface of the iris

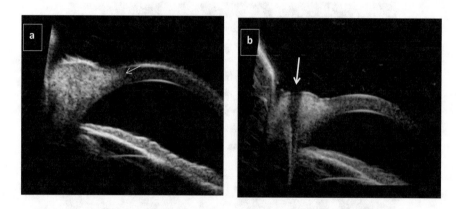

Fig. 5.5 UBM of limbal dermoid **a** infiltration of the corneal stroma (white arrow) with the posterior corneal surface seemed intact **b** With the probe perpendicular on the lesion, it showed the extend of penetration of dermoid reaching the almost the ciliary body where the ciliary body was less clearly visible because of the sound attenuation. Note as well the pathway of low echogenicity inside the limbal dermoid suggestive of the track of hair follicle inside the limbal dermoid (white arrow)

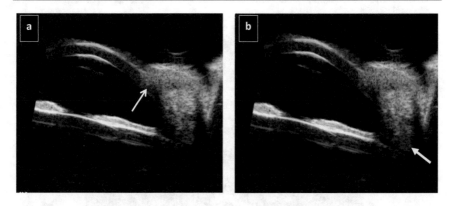

Fig. 5.6 a Limbal dermoid with high reflectivity and almost penetration of all corneal layer (white arrow), **b** intrascleral penetration, (white arrow) with shadowing of the angle and less visibility of the base of the dermoid due to sound attenuation

5.2 Peter's Anomly

Peters' anomaly is a rare developmental abnormality of the anterior segment of the eye and is one of the main causes of congenital corneal opacities. Typically, histopathology of Peters' anomaly shows immature or absent Descemet's membrane and attenuated endothelial cells in the area of the corneal opacity, in addition to thinning or absence of Bowman's membrane and defects in the posterior stroma. Two-thirds of cases are bilateral [2, 8, 21].

Despite the fact that central defect in the corneal endothelium and Descemet's membrane is pathognomonic, about one-half of the patients with Peters' anomaly develop glaucoma. It has been suggested that the increase in intraocular pressure in eyes affected by Peters' anomaly results from incomplete development accompanied by dysfunction of the trabecular meshwork and Schlemm's canal [17, 40, 48, 57]. In addition, cataract may be present and posterior pole malformations such as PFV and colobomas of the disc and retina are common.

More recently, Peters' anomaly was subdivided into two types. Type I is characterized by the central corneal opacity with iridocorneal adhesions, in which the lens may or may not be cataractous, whereas type II is characterized by the central corneal opacity with cataracts or lenticulo-corneal adhesions [16] (Figs. 5.7, 5.8 and 5.9).

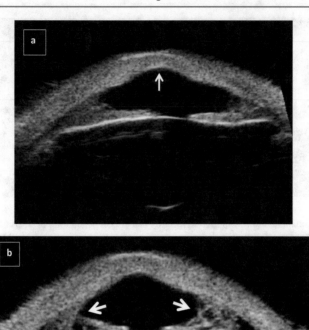

Fig. 5.7 A case of peters' anomly **a** Axial UBM scan showing a central defect in the posterior aspect of the corne(arrow), **b** showing the iridocorneal adhesion (white arrows)

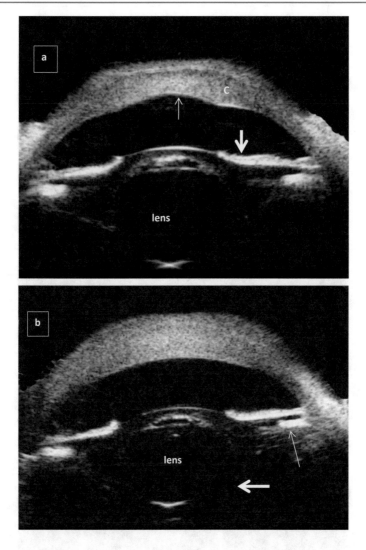

Fig. 5.8 Peter's anomly **a** Axial UBM scan showing a thickened opacified cornea (**c: cornea**) measuring 1.2 mm with shallow anterior chamber measuring 1.6 mm and a defect in the posterior corneal surface (thin arrow), as well as iris hypoplasia (thick arrow) **b** spherical lens (thick arrow) and thin elongated ciliary processes (thin arrow)

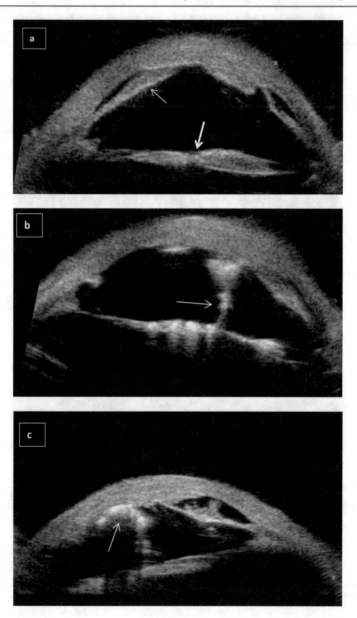

Fig. 5.9 Another case of peters' anomly **a** Axial UBM scan of a thickened opaque cornea with iridocorneal adhesions (thin arrow) and thinned opaque lens (thick arrow), **b** lenticulo-corneal adhesion (arrow), **c** High reflectivity at the lenticulo- corneal adhesion (suggestive of calcification) (arrow)

5.3 Axenfeld-Rieger Syndrome

Axenefeld-Rieger syndrome is an autosomal dominant disease with anterior segment dysgenesis. It is thought to develop from the abnormal migration of neural crest cells. The associated ocular anomalies found are sclerocornea, developmental glaucoma, persistent pupillary membrane, microphthalmos, and the most notable findings are the iris abnormalities that can range from a slight stromal atrophy to extremely minimal presence of iris tissue [4, 10, 12], iridocorneal adhesion, corectopia, polycoria, and posterior embryotoxon [11, 12].

Systemic anomalies associated include facial malformation (telecanthus, maxillary hypoplasia, and flattening of the midface), dental abnormalities (microdontia, oligodontia, hypodontia and adontia), and redundant periumbilical skin. Other

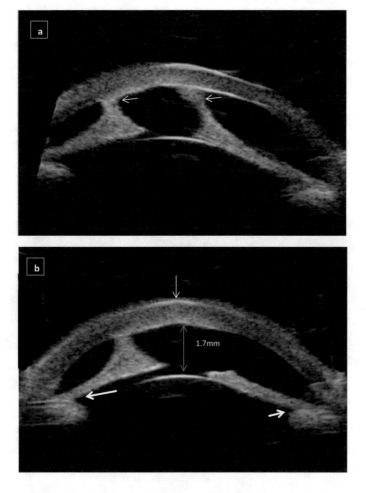

Fig. 5.10 a UBM scans of iridocorneal adhesion at the pupillary margin in the temporal and inferior quadrant (arrows) **b** showing thickened opacified cornea with shallow anterior chamber measuring 1.7 mm, the ciliary body seemed adherent to the posterior iris surface(thick arrows) (The case was diagnosed as Axenfield Rieger syndrome)

uncommon systemic features include congenital heart disease, hearing loss, and growth retardation [18] (Fig. 5.10).

5.4 Aniridia

Aniridia is absence of an iris, which can be divided into hereditary and sporadic forms [34, 37]

*Hereditary aniridia is commonly inherited in an autosomal-dominant manner.

*Classic aniridia is usually accompanied by a variety of ocular anomalies including

(A) keratopathy: Significant cornea opacification may occasionally be the initial manifestation of aniridia.
(B) Lens opacity (cataract): Lens opacities develop in 50% to 85% of the patients usually during the first two decades of life.
(C) Ectopia lentis has been reported in up to 56% of patients with aniridia.
(D) Hypoplastic ciliary processes and anterior inclination of the ciliary processes.
(E) Juvenile-onset glaucoma, foveal hypoplasia and optic nerve hypoplasia.
(F) Pendular nystagmus is present in the majority of aniridias. Iris remnants or a small iris stump can cover the anterior chamber angle forming anterior synechia [35]. Aniridia can also occur as part of the WAGR syndrome (including Wilms tumor, aniridia, genitourinary anomalies and retardation) or Gillespie syndrome (including partial aniridia, ataxia, and intellectual disability) [19, 36] (Figs. 5.11, 5.12, 5.13 and 5.14).

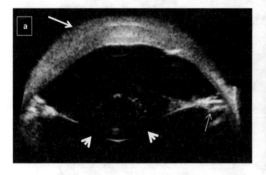
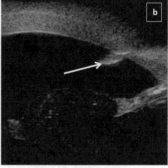

Fig. 5.11 A case of aniridia **a** Axial UBM scan with thickened opaque cornea denoting Keratopathy (white arrow), with aniridia, thin elongated ciliary body(thin arrows) and opaque lens (short arrows) **b** Iris stump closing the angle (arrow)

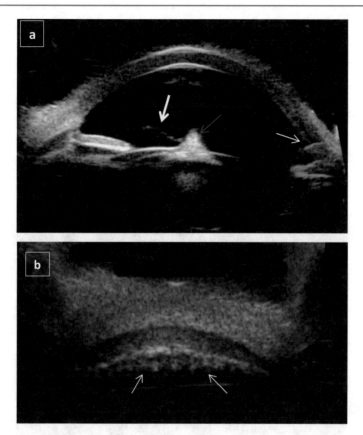

Fig. 5.12 **a** A case of partial aniridia in the temporal and inferior quadrant with iris stump (thin arrow) and anterior lenticonus(red arrow), and persistent pupillary membrane(thick arrow), **b** Transverse scan showing the hypoplastic ciliary processes (arrows)

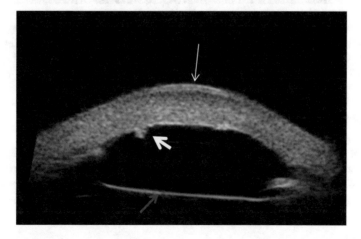

Fig. 5.13 A case of aniridia with iris stump (thick arrow) and Keratopathy (thin arrow),the patient is aphakic with opacified posterior capsule (red arrow)

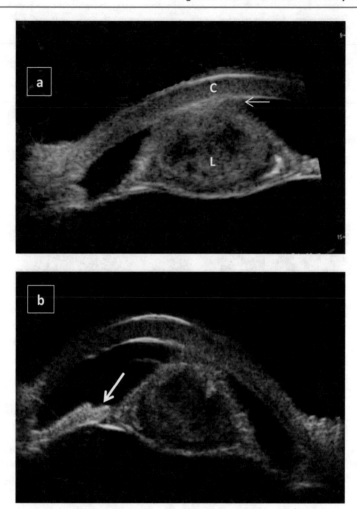

Fig. 5.14 **a** A case of partial aniridia in the temporal and inferior quadrant with cataract of ectopia lentis and lenticulo-corneal adhesion (white arrow), **b** showing bifurcation at the pupillary edge of the iris at the nasal quadrant (white arrow). (C: cornea- L: lens)

5.5   Posterior Lenticonus

Posterior lenticonus is a congenital defect, which is a sporadic and unilateral in most cases. It is a localized, well-demarcated bulging of the posterior capsule and cortex of the lens, where its pathogenesis is not known. Bilateral cases have been reported and are generally associated with family history [60] (Figs. 5.15 and 5.16).

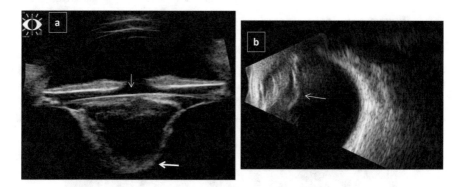

Fig. 5.15 **a** Axial UBM scan showing posterior lenticonus (thick arrow) with opacified lens and flat anterior capsule (thin arrow), **b** B-scan showing the protrusion of the posterior capsule (white arrow)

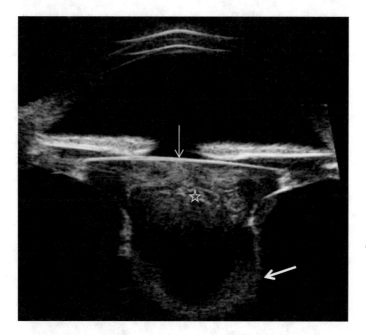

Fig. 5.16 Another case with posterior lenticonus (thick arrow) with opacified lens (star) and flat anterior capsule (thin arrow)

5.6 Persistent Fetal Vasculature (PFV)

Persistent fetal vasculature is a congenital developmental disorder that occurs when the vascular structures present during the development of the eye fail to regress as they should. It is present at birth, predominantly unilateral in 90% of the cases. It can be purely anterior, posterior or combined. It has a characteristic clinical appearance of localized cataract and prominent ciliary processes which are features of the anterior form [13, 28, 45].

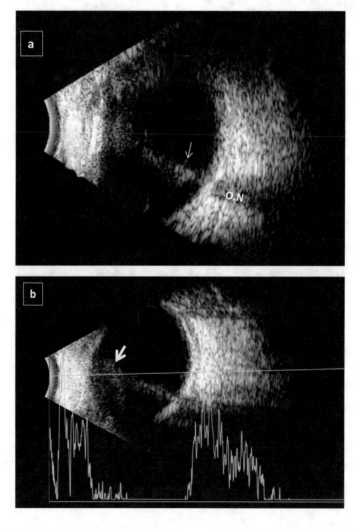

Fig. 5.17 PFV **a** Longitudnal scan showing a fine membrane of low echogenicity (white arrow) extending from anterior aspect of the eye to the optic nerve (O.N)posteriorly, **b** showing the retrolental membrane (thick arrow) with low reflectivity in A-scan (thin arrow)

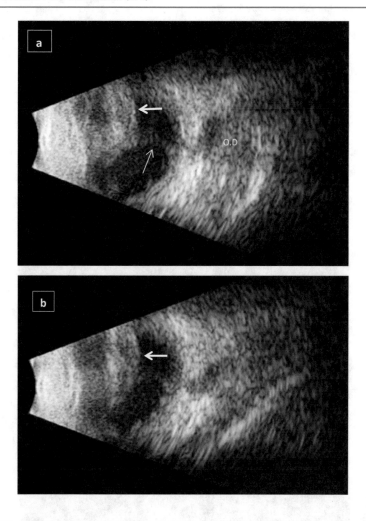

Fig. 5.18 **a** Axial scan showing a fine membrane (PFV) (thin arrow) extending from the optic nerve posteriorly to a thick band in the retrolental space (thick arrows) in (**a** and **b**), Note the short axial length measuring ±15.00 mm compared to the fellow eye with an axial length of 20.00 mm

The posterior PFV echography appears as a vitreous band of variable reflectivity extending from the lens to the optic disc. It is advised to increase the gain settings to detect a low reflective strand, however, the entire extent of the vitreous band may not be visible in all cases. The lens is often thin with irregular posterior capsule. PFV can cause peripapillary tractional retinal detachments [46].

The axial length of the affected eye shows a shorter than normal globe. Therefore, it is important to compare axial lengths in an eye with unilateral cataract, although it may be normal in some patient.

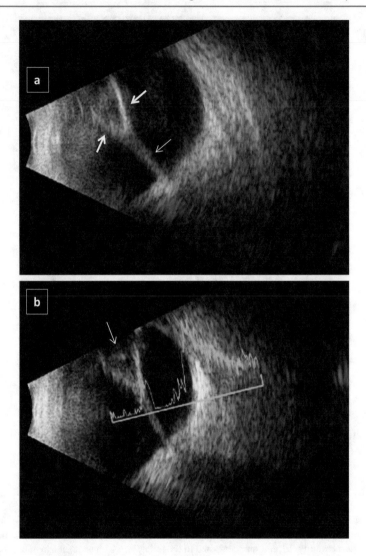

Fig. 5.19 a Longitudinal scan of a case of thick PFV (thin arrow). Note the insertion of the bifurcation of the membrane anteriorly(thick arrows), **b** longitudinal scan exposing the lens (arrow) anteriorly showing the insertion of the PFV at the back of the irregular shape of the opaque lens,Note the moderate amplitude in A-scan of the PFV

A thick band secondary to PFV can be confused with tightly closed funnel-shaped retinal detachment, Identification of small area of traction posteriorly or the anterior attachment of the thick band can help in differentiation [57] (Figs. 5.17, 5.18, 5.19, 5.20, 5.21 and 5.22).

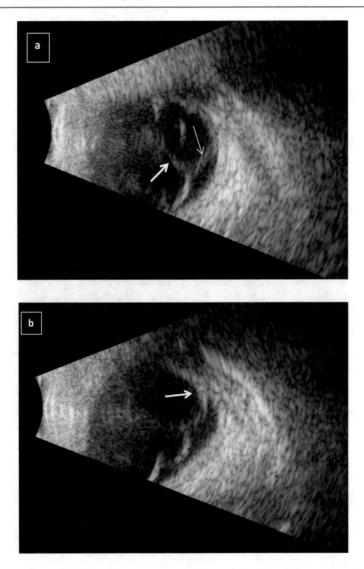

Fig. 5.20 A case of PFV (thick arrow) causing traction retinal detachment, **a** Transverse scan of central traction retinal detachment (thin arrow) by the PFV, **b** Longitudinal scan showing the extension of the retinal detachment anteriorly (white arrow)

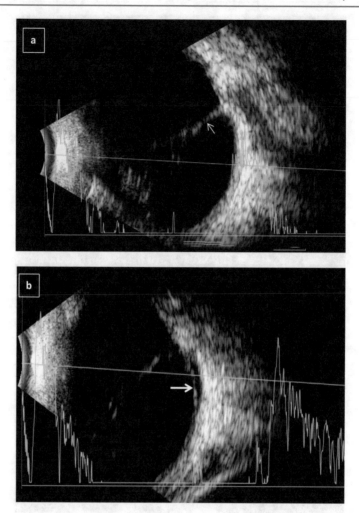

Fig. 5.21 A case of PFV **a** A visible membrane posteriorly with decreased its echogenicity anteriorly (white arrow) **b** showing localized traction retinal detachment temporal to the optic disc (white arrow)

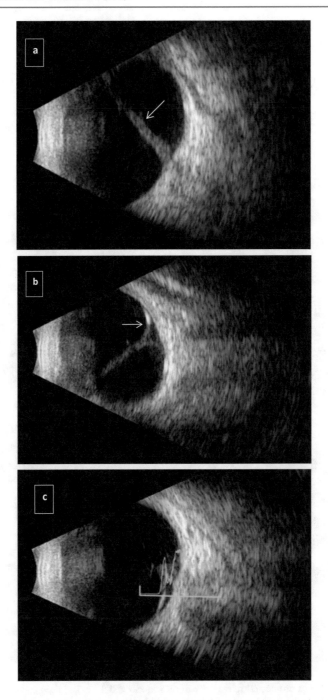

Fig. 5.22 a A longitudnal scan showing thick PFV (white arrow), **b** and **c** paraaxial scan and longitudnal scan with juxtapapillary traction retinal detachment (tent shape) (white arrow) caused by the PFV, Note the high reflectivity of the retina in the superimposed A-scan in (**c**)

5.7 Retinopathy of Prematurity (ROP)

Retinopathy of prematurity (ROP) usually affects low birth weight premature infants, with gestational age less than 32 weeks and birth weight less than 1500 g, It is typically a bilateral condition, which is present in normal or smaller sized eye. It occurs due to proliferation of abnormal blood vessels in the peripheral fundus in response to incomplete vascularization of the peripheral retina and exposure to oxygen [51].

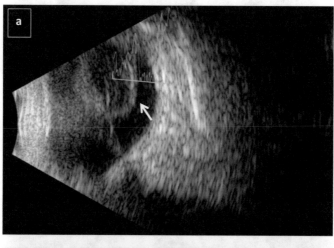

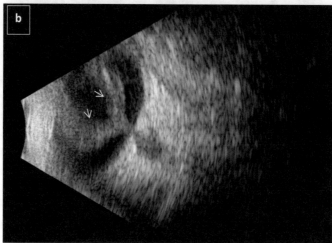

Fig. 5.23 A case of bilateral retinopathy of prematurity (ROP) **a** The right eye showing closed funnel shaped retinal detachment, with large retinal loop anteriorly (white arrow). **b** the Left eye showing open funnel retinal detachment (arrows) with thickened retinal leaves, Note the small size of the eye with an axial length of 17.00 mm bilaterally

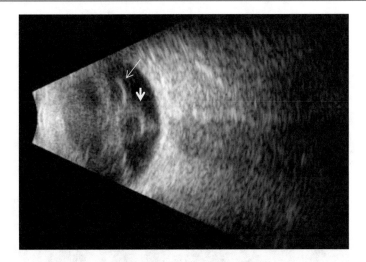

Fig. 5.24 A case of ROP, Axial scan showing a funnel-shaped retinal detachment with an open funnel posteriorly (thick white arrow), as well as formation of an anterior retinal loop (thin white arrow). Note the accumulation of echoes in the anterior part suggesting the presence of preretinal fibrous tissue (red arrow)

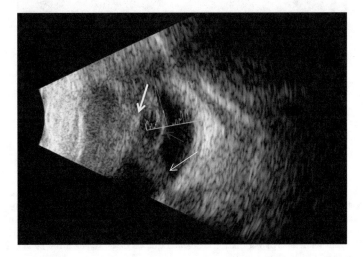

Fig. 5.25 ROP, Longitudinal scan showing funnel shaped retinal detachment with tightly closed funnel posteriorly (white arrow), Note The retrolental space showing densely packed echoes suggestive of fibrous tissue (thick white arrow), Note as well the high reflectivity of the peripheral retinal loop(red arrow)

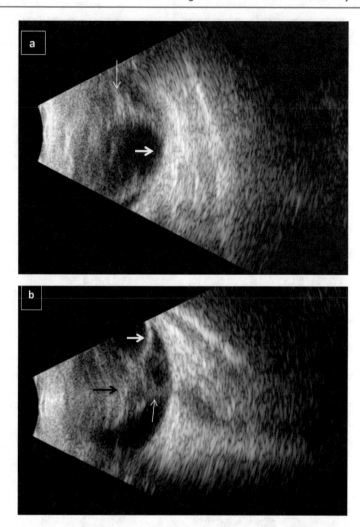

Fig. 5.26 ROP with stage 4 in the right eye and stage 5 in the Left eye **a** Longitudnal scan of the right eye showing peripheral retinal detachment with thickened anterior retina, denoting presence of preretinal fibrous tissue (thin arrow), with central retina in place (thick arrow). **b** Axial scan of the Left eye of the same paient showing total funnel retinal detachment with tightly closed funnel posteriorly (thin white arrow) with dense retrolental fibrous tissue (black arrow) and evidence of large retinal loop (thick white arrow)

The ultrasound features in the early stages of ROP appear as an acoustic reflex suggestive of a ridge in the region between the ciliary body and the equator (stage 2) is seen, while stage 3 is described as elevation or layer separation in this anterior retinal ridge region [29]

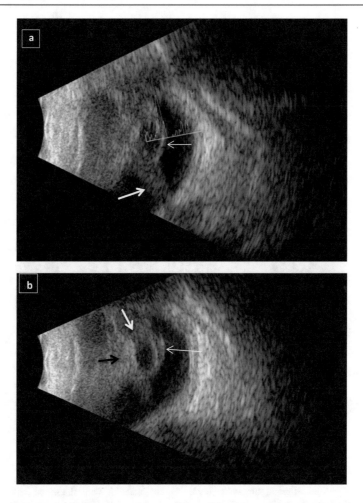

Fig. 5.27 ROP **a** Longitudnal scan showing closed funnel retinal detachment (thick white arrow) with formation of retinal loop (thin arrow) which is more demonstrated in (**b**) a longitudnal scan revealing the anterior retina showing the retinal loop with the periretinal fibrous tissue attached to it (thick white arrow), note the retrolental fibrous tissue (black arrow)

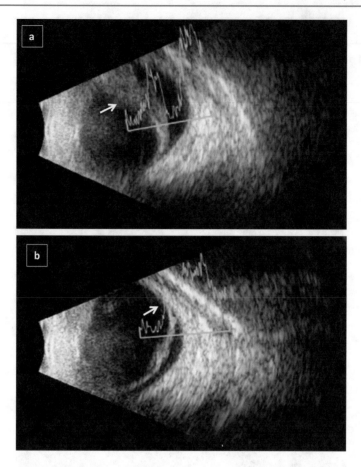

Fig. 5.28 ROP stage 4B, with subtotal retinal detachment **a** Longitudinal scan showing retinal detachment in the temporal quadrant (involving the macula) with thickened retinal leaves anteriorly denoting the presence of periretinal fibrous tissue attached to the retina (white arrow). **b** Transverse scan of the temporal quadrant showing the retina attached in the temporal quadrant superiorly (white arrow)

In advanced cases as in Stage 4 there is a subtotal retinal detachment, which is sub divided into Partial retinal detachment not involving the fovea (stage 4A) and Partial retinal detachment involving the fovea (stage 4B), where in stage 5 the retina is extensively detached in a funnel-shaped appearance with the peripheral retina frequently having a loops or trough-like appearance as a result of traction by these dense retrolental membranes [3, 52, 56, 61].

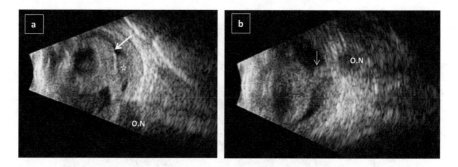

Fig. 5.29 ROP **a** longitudinal B-scan of the right eye showing retinal detachment with thickened retina (white arrow) due to periretinal fibrous tissue and subretinal echoes of subretinal hemorrhage (star) **b** Axial B-scan showing total funnel retinal detachment with open funnel anteriorly (red arrows) and closed funnel posteriorly (white arrow) (O.N: optic nerve)

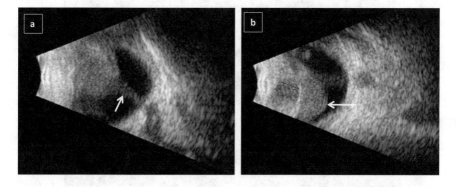

Fig. 5.30 ROP **a** longitudinal B-scan of the Left eye of the same patient showing a closed funnel retinal detachment (white arrow) with retrolental fibrous tissue. **b** Axial B scan showing peripheral retinal loop (white arrow) with the retrolental fibrous tissue, Note the lens (red arrow)

It is important to identify the exact configuration of the funnel retinal detachment (open or closed, either anteriorly, posteriorly or both), where there is usually an anterior narrowing of the funnel retina before a posterior narrowing. So it is important to identify those cases with open posterior configurations, because these are more easily approached surgically and often have more hope for restoration of some vision than do eyes with closed posterior funnels, in which the retina often cannot be flattened [31, 55]. The detection of subretinal echoes which could be blood or cholesterol signifies a poor prognosis (Figs. 5.23, 5.24, 5.25, 5.26, 5.27, 5.28, 5.29 and 5.30).

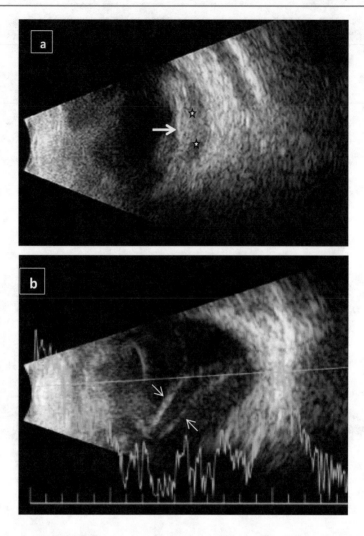

Fig. 5.31 Coats' disease **a** Transverse scan showing exudative retinal detachment (white arrow) with dense echoes in the subretinal space(stars), **b** Paraxial scan showing retinoschesis (white arrows)with multiple echoes of low echogenicity between the retinal layers. No evidence of mass lesion

5.8 Coats Disease

Coats' disease is a common cause of exudative retinal detachment in childhood. It is a retinal vascular disorder characterized by telangiectasia, intraretinal exudation, and exudative retinal detachment [24, 32]. It is unilateral in the majority of cases

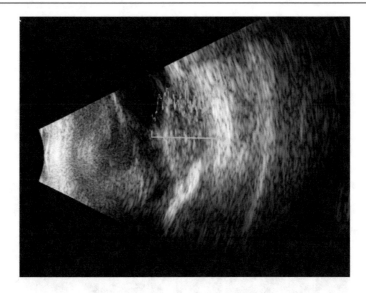

Fig. 5.32 B-scan of a case of Coats' with exudative retinal detachment and medium to high reflective spikes of the subretinal echoes (denoting cholesterol)

and considered as important cause of leukokoria and hence a differential diagnosis for retinoblastoma, Ultrasound is indicated to confirm the diagnosis and rule out retinoblastoma (Figs. 5.31, 5.32, and 5.33).

Coats' disease has different stages depending on how it is affecting the retinal and its capillaries. At the early stages, it's characterized by being localized. At advanced stages, total retinal detachment is more likely to occur, which can even touch the lens [53, 54]. Visualisation of the fundus is often hampered by the high, closed funnel retinal detachment and other factors such as corneal oedema, posterior synaechiae and retrolental (cyclitic) membrane [25]. The vascular abnormalities associated with Coats' disease most frequently occur superotemporally, and exudative retinal detachments can occur as the disease progresses [23, 26, 43]

Echographic appearance however becomes more diagnostic as the disease advances and consists of:

*Narrow or closed funnel-shaped retinal detachment with looping of the peripheral retina, with poor retinal mobility on kinetic scan.

*Dense, dispersed, low to medium reflective subretinal (cholesterol) opacities exhibiting constant slow convection movement.

*Absence of solid mass lesion with no evidence of calcium foci.

*Calcification of the detached retina, and other ocular tissues, may also be encountered in long standing Coats' disease [25].

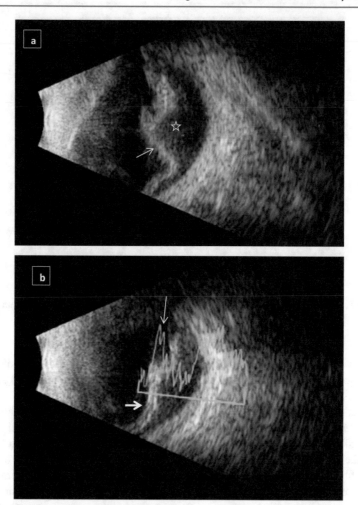

Fig. 5.33 **a** A case of Coats' disease with exudative retinal detachment and thickened retina (white arrow) with multiple echoes of low to moderate echoegenicity in the subretinal space(star), **b** Evidence of retinal layers separation (thick arrow), note the double high spikes (thin arrow) of retinal layer in the superimposed A-scan

5.9 Retinoblastoma

Retinoblastoma is a rare form of eye cancer that usually develops in early child-hood, typically before the age of 5 years. While leukocoria is the most common presenting symptom of retinoblastoma, other less common symptoms have been observed such as strabismus, decreased vision and ocular inflammation [9, 44].

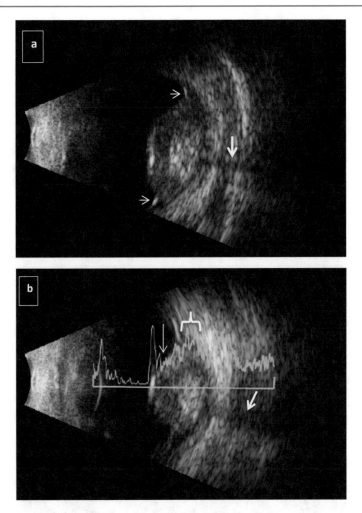

Fig. 5.34 Endophytic retinoblastoma: **a** Dome-shaped retinal mass with multiple echoes of high echogenicity inside the mass consistent with calcification (red arrow) which cause shadowing to the orbital tissue posteriorly (white arrow), with evidence of retinal detachment at the edges of the tumour (short white arrows) **b** showing the superimposed A-scan with low reflectivity of the tumour (thin white arrow) and increased reflectivity of the calcification (brace)with shadowing to the orbital tissue posterior to the tumour (white arrow)

At its earliest clinical stage, retinoblastoma appears as a flat transparent to slightly whitish colored lesion in the sensory retina. As the tumor enlarges, it loses its transparency and takes on a creamy yellow to whitish coloration with foci of chalk-like calcification. As it grows further beyond the boundary of the sensory retina, retinoblastoma will typically follow either an endophytic or exophytic growth pattern [33, 59]

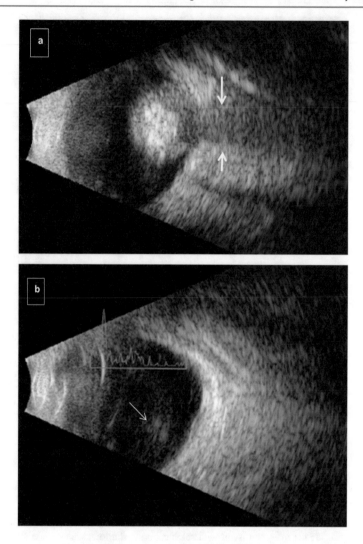

Fig. 5.35 Endophytic retinoblastoma: **a** Dome-shaped retinal mass close to the optic disc (3.50 mm nasal to the optic disc) with a large area of calcification inside the tumour of high echogenicty causing shadowing to the orbital tissue posteriorly (white arrow) **b** transverse scan of another quadrant showing echoes of moderate echogenicity in the vitreous cavity denoting vitreous cells (white arrow)

Endophytic retinoblastomas grow from the retina inward towards the vitreous cavity. Vitreous seeding from these friable tumors as well as anterior chamber involvement can simulate endophthalmitis and other inflammatory conditions [39] (Figs. 5.34 and 5.35).

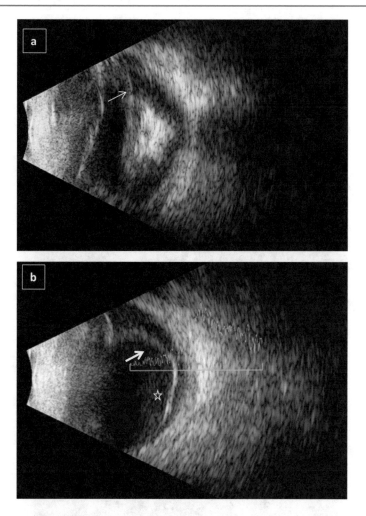

Fig. 5.36 Exophytic retinoblastoma **a** Axial scan of a large retinoblastoma in the subretinal space with retinal detachment displaced behined the lens (white arrow), and dense calcification(red arrows), **b** longitudinal scan exposing the extension of the retinal detachment in other quadrants with evidence of vitreous cells (star)

Exophytic retinoblastomas grow from the retina outward into the subretinal space and can cause exudative retinal detachment, sometimes displacing the retina anteriorly behind the lens [39] (Fig. 5.36).

Ultrasonography is helpful in confirming the diagnosis of retinoblastoma and in differentiating the disease from other causes of leukocoria. B-scan ultrasonography typically displays a rounded or dome-shaped or irregular intraocular mass. Mildly elevated and diffuse lesions have also been reported, however, large tumors are highly irregular and heterogeneous in texture. When a significant degree of

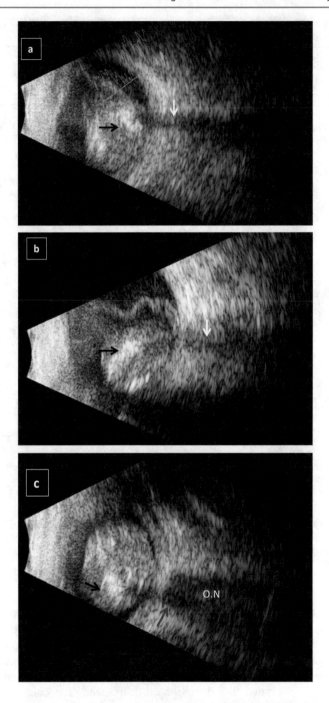

Fig. 5.37 a and **b** Large retinoblastoma with dense calcification (black arrows) causing shadowing to the orbital tissue (white arrows), with evidence of thick retinal detachment)(red arrow in B) and vitreous cells, **c** Axial scan of the retinoblastoma reaching the optic nerve (O.N) with calcification (black arrow) causing shadowing at the edge of the optic nerve (red arrow)

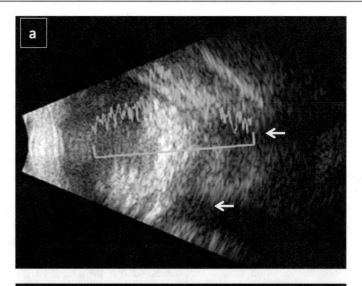

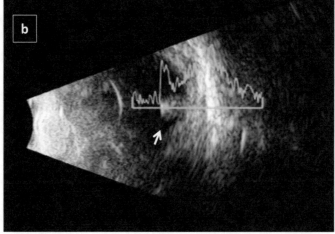

Fig. 5.38 **a** Right eye showing irregular retinoblastoma with large broad calcification with high amplitude in A-scan, causing multiple area of shadowing (white arrows) to the orbital tissue, **b** B-scan of the Lt eye showing a small retinoblastoma (white arrow) in the inferonasal quadrant anteriorly

calcification is present, shadowing of the adjacent sclera and orbit occurs [47, 49] (Figs. 5.37 and 5.38).

On A-scan, the internal reflectivity of these lesions varies in accordance to the degree of calcification within the tumor. Non-calcified tumors exhibit low to medium internal reflectivity, whereas calcified lesions demonstrate high internal reflectivity.

Retinoblastoma may spread either by hematogenous dissemination or by direct extension either through the bulbar wall into the orbit or via the optic nerve and its meningeal sheath [22, 39, 50], When extraocular extension is present, invasion of the optic nerve is the most common route.

5.10 Coloboma

Colobomas result from a failure of the embryonic fissure to close and are characteristically located in the inferior-nasal part of the fundus. Eyes with coloboma are likely to be microphthalmic. Complete or partial colobomas may occur anywhere along the fusion lines extending from the iris margin to the optic disc [14, 42]

Histologically, the colobomatous area is deficient in normal choroid, retinal pigment epithelium (RPE), and the retina. The neurosensory retina continues as the intercalary membrane (ICM) in the area of coloboma [6, 27]. Breaks in the intercalary membrane stretched across the coloboma are the cause of most retinal detachments associated with choroidal colobomas [15] (Figs. 5.39 and 5.40).

A coloboma of the choroid appears in ultrasonography as an excavation of varying depth involving the choroid, optic disc or both. The contour of the coloboma may be either smooth or have an outpouching, while the edge is typically overhanging and sharp or shelved, which helps distinguish it from a posterior staphyloma, which has a smooth edge [58] (Figs. 5.41, 5.42 and 5.43).

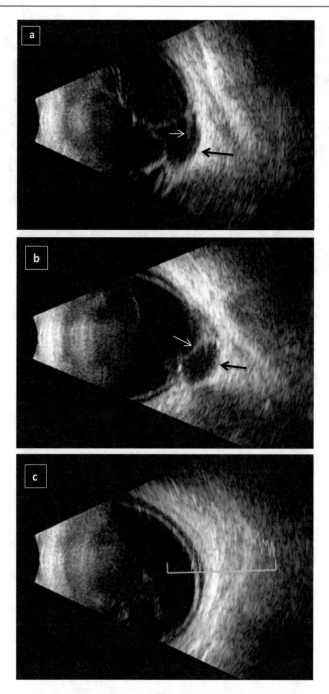

Fig. 5.39 a B-scan of choroidal coloboma (black arrows) with total retinal detachment. Note the taut membranes extending from the base of the coloboma to the detached retina (white arrow), **b** longitudinal scan showing the choroidal coloboma with detached ICM (white arow), **c** showing the extension of the retinal detachment

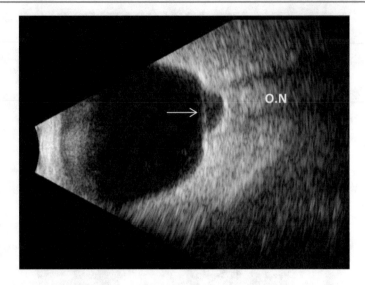

Fig. 5.40 B scan image of an eye with a choroidal coloboma around the optic disc. A moderately reflective membrane is seen stretched across the coloboma, which represents a detached intercalary membrane (white arrow)

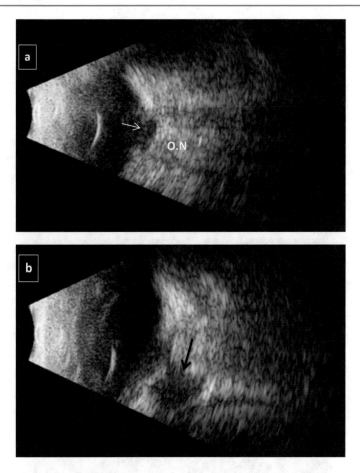

Fig. 5.41   a A large coloboma of the choroid involving the optic disc area (white arrow) **b** Cystic outpouching at the lower border of the coloboma (black arrow)

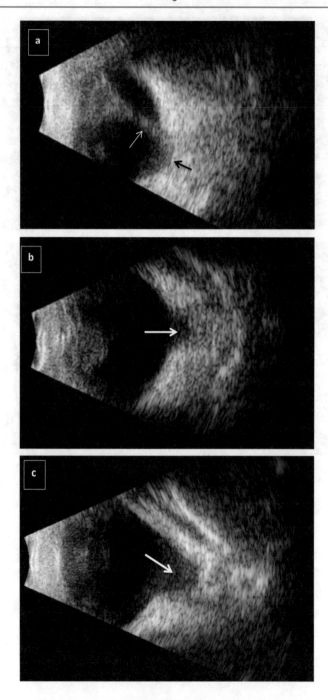

Fig. 5.42 B-scan images of optic nerve coloboma with persistent fetal vasculature (PFV), **a** Longitudnal scan exposing the PFV (white arrow) insertion to the edge of the optic nerve coloboma (black arrow) and to the lens anteriorly, **b** and **c** different scans of the same patient exposing the depth of the coloboma (white arrows)

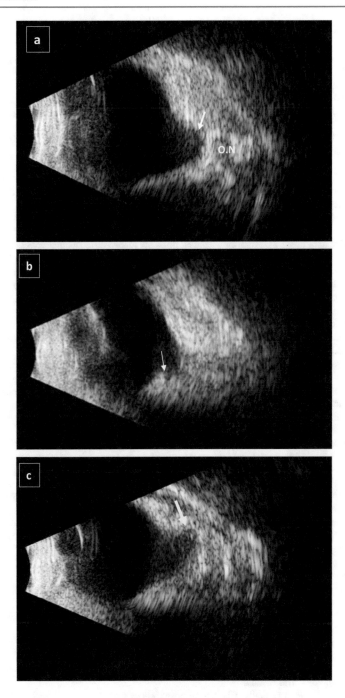

Fig. 5.43 Coloboma of the optic disc and choroid. Different B scan images of the same patient exposing **a** coloboma of the optic disc (arrow) **b** and **c** coloboma of adjacent choroid (white arrows) and its depth. (O.N: optic nerve)

References

1. Schulze RR. Limbal dermoid tumor with intraocular extension. Arch Ophthalmol. 1966;75.
2. Ozeki H, et al. Ocular and systemic features of Peters' anomaly. Graefe's Arch Clin Exp Ophthalmol. 2000;238(10):833–9.
3. Dou G-R, et al. Demographic profile and ocular characteristics of stage 5 retinopathy of prematurity at a referral center in Northwest China: implications for implementation. BMC Ophthalmol. 2018;18(1):1–9.
4. Ozeki H, et al. Anomalies associated with Axenfeld-Rieger syndrome. Graefes Arch Clin Exp Ophthalmol. 1999;237(9):730–4.
5. Hoops JP, et al. Preoperative evaluation of limbal dermoids using high-resolution biomicroscopy. Graefe's Arch Clin Exp Ophthalmol. 2001;239(6):459–61.
6. Schubert HD. Schisis-like rhegmatogenous retinal detachment associated with choroidal colobomas. Graefes Arch Clin Exp Ophthalmol. 1995;233(2):74–9.
7. Nevares RL, Mulliken JB, Robb RM. Ocular dermoids. Plast Reconstr Surg. 1988;82(6):959–64.
8. Mireskandari K, et al. Anterior segment imaging in pediatric ophthalmology. J. Cataract Refract Surg. 2011;37(12):2201–10.
9. Subha L, Arun Subhash Reddy R. A clinical study of retinoblastoma. J Pharmacy Bioallied Sci. 2015;7(Suppl 1):S2.
10. Guerriero S, et al. Combined aniridia ring implantation and cataract surgery in an Axenfeld–Rieger syndrome: a UBM report. Eye Contact Lens. 2011;37(1):45–7.
11. Wang X, et al. Mutation survey of candidate genes and genotype–phenotype analysis in 20 Southeastern Chinese patients with Axenfeld–Rieger syndrome. Curr Eye Res. 2018;43 (11):1334–41.
12. Chang TC, et al. Axenfeld-Rieger syndrome: new perspectives. Br J Ophthalmol. 2012;96 (3):318–22.
13. Aponte EP, et al. A novel NDP mutation in an infant with unilateral persistent fetal vasculature and retinal vasculopathy. Ophthalmic Genet. 2009;30(2):99–102.
14. Toker E, et al. Colobomatous macrophthalmia with microcornea syndrome: report of a new pedigree. Am J Med Genet Part A. 2003;121(1):25–30.
15. Hanneken A, de Juan Jr E, McCuen II BW. The management of retinal detachments associated with choroidal colobomas by vitreous surgery. Am J Ophthalmol. 1991;111 (3):271–5.
16. Ni W, et al. A novel histopathologic finding in the Descemet's membrane of a patient with Peters Anomaly: a case-report and literature review. BMC Ophthalmol. 2015;15(1):1–5.
17. Todorova MG, et al. Anterior segment dysgenesis associated with Williams-Beuren syndrome: a case report and review of the literature. BMC Ophthalmol. 2014;14(1):1–5.
18. Singh S, et al. Axenfeld Rieger syndrome: a rare developmental disorder. The Official Sci J Delhi Ophthalmol Soc. 2015;24(4):263–5.
19. Lin Y, et al. Two paired box 6 mutations identified in Chinese patients with classic congenital aniridia and cataract. Mol Med Rep. 2018;18(5):4439–45.
20. Shigeyasu C, et al. Clinical features of anterior segment dysgenesis associated with congenital corneal opacities. Cornea 2012;31(3):293–8.
21. Nischal KK, et al. Clinicopathological correlation of congenital corneal opacification using ultrasound biomicroscopy. Br J Ophthalmol. 2002;86(1):62–9.
22. Abdu L, Sani M. Clinicopathological pattern and management of retinoblastoma in Kano, Nigeria. Ann Afr Med. 2011;10(3).
23. Ali FS, Do DV, Haller JA. Coats' Disease and Retinal Telangiectasia, Elsevier 2018; Ophthalmology fifth edition.
24. Budning AS, Heon E, Gallie BL. Visual prognosis of Coats' disease. J Am Assoc Pediatric Ophthalmol Strabismus. 1998;2(6):356–9.

25. Atta HR, Watson NJ. Echographic diagnosis of advanced Coats' disease. Eye. 1992;6(1):80–5.
26. Nikolas JS, Shields CL, Haller JA. Coats Disease, Retina 5th Edition, 2012.
27. Gopal L, et al. A clinical and optical coherence tomography study of the margins of choroidal colobomas. Ophthalmology 2007;114(3):571–80.
28. Hu A, et al. Combined persistent fetal vasculature: a classification based on high-resolution B-mode ultrasound and color Doppler imaging. Ophthalmology 2016;123(1):19–25.
29. Jokl DH, et al. Is there a role for high-frequency ultrasonography in clinical staging of retinopathy of prematurity? J Pediatric Ophthalmol Strabismus 2006;43(1):31–5.
30. Arora R, Jain V, Mehta D. Deep lamellar keratoplasty in corneal dermoid. Eye. 2005;19(8):920–1.
31. Machemer R. Description and pathogenesis of late stages of retinopathy of prematurity. Ophthalmology. 1985;92(8):1000–4.
32. Ghorbanian S, Jaulim A, Chatziralli IP. Diagnosis and treatment of coats' disease: a review of the literature. Ophthalmologica. 2012;227(4):175–82.
33. Abramson DAVIDH. The diagnosis of retinoblastoma. Bull New York Acad Med. 1988;64(4):283.
34. Nelson LB, et al. Aniridia. A review. Survey Ophthalmol. 1984;28(6):621–42.
35. Viestenz A, et al. Clinical anatomy of the anterior chamber angle in congenital aniridia and consequences for trabeculotomy/cyclophotocoagulation. Clin Anat. 2018;31(1):64–7.
36. Moosajee M, Melanie H, Moore AT. PAX6-related aniridia. (2018).
37. Okamoto F, et al. Ultrasound biomicroscopic findings in aniridia. Am J Ophthalmol. 2004;137(5):858–62.
38. Cennamo G, et al. Evaluation of morning glory syndrome with spectral optical coherence tomography and echography. Ophthalmology 2010;117(6):1269–73.
39. de Graaf P, et al. Guidelines for imaging retinoblastoma: imaging principles and MRI standardization. Pediatric Radiol. 2012;42(1):2–14.
40. Siebelmann S, et al. Intraoperative optical coherence tomography in children with anterior segment anomalies. Ophthalmology 2015;122(12):2582–4.
41. Pirouzian A. Management of pediatric corneal limbal dermoids. Clin Ophthalmol (Auckland, NZ). 2013;7:607.
42. Magni R, Pierro L, Brancato R. Microphthalmos with colobomatous orbital cyst in trisomy 13. Ophthalmic Paediatr Genet. 1991;12(1):39–42.
43. Buzzard AK, Linklater DR. Pediatric retinal detachment due to Coats' Disease diagnosed with bedside emergency department ultrasound. J Emerg Med. 2009;37(4):390–2.
44. Castillo Jr, Bienvenido V, Kaufman L. Pediatric tumors of the eye and orbit. Pediatric Clinics North Am. 2003;50(1):149–72.
45. Goldberg MF. Persistent fetal vasculature (PFV): an integrated interpretation of signs and symptoms associated with persistent hyperplastic primary vitreous (PHPV) LIV Edward Jackson Memorial Lecture. Am J Ophthalmol. 1997;124(5):587–626.
46. Promelle V, Bryselbout S, Milazzo S. Visual prognosis of posterior and combined persistent fetal vasculature. Eur J Ophthalmol. 2020;30(2):284–8.
47. Giacalone M, Mastrangelo G, Parri N. Point-of-care ultrasound diagnosis of retinoblastoma in the emergency department. Pediatr Emerg Care. 2018;34(8):599–601.
48. Sagara T, et al. Pupillary block in Peters' anomaly. Invest Ophthalmol Vis Sci. 2007;48(13):4350–4350.
49. Soni HC, et al. Pictorial essay: USG of retinoblastoma. Indian J Radiol Imaging. 2006;16(4):657.
50. Ray A, Gombos DS. Retinoblastoma: an overview. The Indian Journal of Pediatrics. 2012;79(7):916–21.
51. Velez-Montoya R, et al. Intraocular and systemic levels of vascular endothelial growth factor in advanced cases of retinopathy of prematurity. Clin Ophthalmol (Auckland, NZ) 2010;4:947.

52. Shapiro MJ, Alpert J, Pandit RT. Tent-shaped retinal detachments in retinopathy of prematurity. Retina. 2006;26(7):S32–7.
53. Li S, et al. The effects of a treatment combination of anti-VEGF injections, laser coagulation and cryotherapy on patients with type 3 Coat's disease. BMC Ophthalmol. 2017;17(1):1–7.
54. Bansal S, Niladri S, Woon WH. The management of "Coats' Response" in a patient with X-linked retinitis pigmentosa—a case report. ISRN Surg. 2011;2011.
55. de Juan Jr E, Shields S, Machemer R. The role of ultrasound in the management of retinopathy of prematurity. Ophthalmology 1988;95(7):884–8.
56. Shapiro DR, Stone RD. Ultrasonic characteristics of retinopathy of prematurity presenting with leukokoria. Arch Ophthalmol. 1985;103(11):1690–2.
57. Byrne SF, Green RL. Ultrasound of the eye and orbit. 2nd ed. St. Louis: Mosby, Inc.; 2002.
58. Bhende M, Kamat H, Krishna T, Shantha B, Sen P, Khetan V, Pradeep S. Atlas of Ophthalmic Ultrasound And Ultrasound Biomicroscopy, Second Edition;2013. ISBN 978-93-5090-535-7.
59. Singh AD, Lorek BH. Ophthalmic Ultrasonography E-Book: Expert Consult-Online and Print. Elsevier Health Sciences;2011.
60. Khokhar S, et al. Posterior lenticonus with persistent fetal vasculature. Indian J Ophthalmol. 2018;66(9):1335.
61. Shah PK, et al. Retinopathy of prematurity: past, present and future. World J Clin Pediatr. 2016;5(1):35.

Ocular Tumors

6

6.1 Anterior Segment Tumors

UBM is considered as the gold standard in the imaging of anterior segment tumors. It provides clear visualization of even the smallest anterior segment lesions, especially in areas inaccessible to visualization in a basic ophthalmological examination. UBM enables the assessment of tumor parameters such as size, location, infiltration of surrounding structures and growth rate, which allows improved classification and ability to determine ciliary body involvement.

Moreover, it helps in the assessment of tumor features such as internal reflectivity, hyper or hypo-echoic patterns suggestive of vascular and cystic areas. These important diagnostic and prognostic parameters provide key information about the appropriate management and surgical approach, if indicated [39].

6.1.1 Iris Lesions

a) Iris Cysts

Primary Neuroepithelial Cysts: Usually bilateral or multiloculated, highly reflective, smooth cyst wall, with no solid component.

Implantation Cysts: Diffuse/dense internal echoes, with site of origin of the cyst may be demonstrated, such as limbal or corneal wound.

Spontaneously occurring cysts are usually found in relationship to the iris or ciliary body. These cysts are most commonly found at the iridociliary junction [22], but can be found at other locations related to the iris and iris epithelium.

Iridociliary cysts usually present as small localized elevations of the iris, displays these lesions as thin-walled cysts, with no internal reflectivity, and occasional multiloculations. The total lack of internal reflectivity indicates a fluid-filled cyst and this feature eliminates any possibility of confusion with a solid lesion [1] (Figs. 6.1 and 6.2).

R. Abbas, *Ophthalmic Ultrasonography and Ultrasound Biomicroscopy*,
https://doi.org/10.1007/978-3-030-76979-6_6

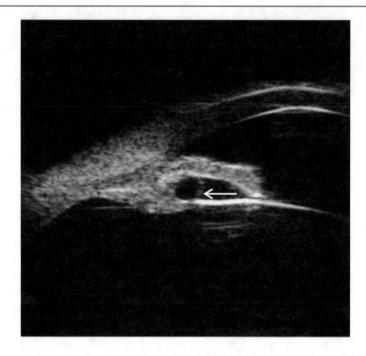

Fig. 6.1 Longitudinal UBM scan of an iridociliary cyst (arrow) in the iridociliary junction causing elevation of the iris

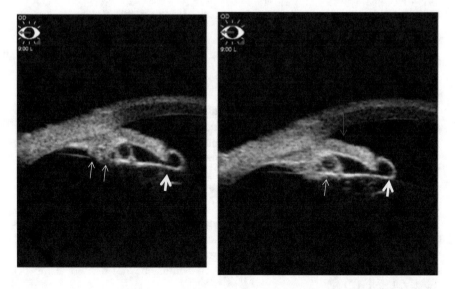

Fig. 6.2 Multiple thick walled, multiloculated cysts in the iridocilary junction (thin arrows) causing elevation of the iris (red arrow). Note the iris cyst at the pupillary margin (thick arrows)

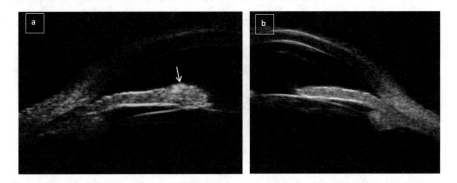

Fig. 6.3 Iris nevus, **a** longitudinal scans showing thickening of the iris at the pupillary margin with increased echogenicity (arrow) of the iris epithelium compared to **b** the normal iris configuration of the same patient at the opposite quadrant)

b) Iris Nevus

Iris nevus are benign lesions with minimal or no growth tendency however, they should be monitored regularly over time for any neoplastic changes. An Iris nevus appears as a solid plaque-like lesion on the anterior iris surface and/or stroma. Iris nevi have more a predilection for the inferior half of the iris, and they are commonly solitary and circumscribed.

Ultrasound biomicroscopic appearance shows a low reflective surface plaque overlying an area of iris thickening. Surface plaques are frequently seen and are often very thin (50–150/μm) [1]. The posterior iris surface flat or smoothly concave. With minor degrees of pupil distortion (Fig. 6.3)

c) Iris Melanoma

Iris melanomas can be variable in their clinical and ultrasonic presentation, On UBM, it appears as a solid irregular iris mass with variable internal reflectivity. Some melanomas show a linear internal reflectivity, while others show uniform reflectivity. This causes irregularity or convex bowing of the posterior iris plane. Involvement of the iris root and disruption of the posterior surface of the iris pigment epithelium are considered signs of metastasis and posterior tumor extension, causing distortion of the surrounding structures. Invasion of the ciliary body typically appears on UBM as an area of reduced reflectivity in continuity with the iris mass [2].

The surface plaque is hyporeflective if the cells are packed (spindle cell type) and hyper-reflective if cells are loosely packed (epithelioid cell type). Also UBM detects internal vascularity reliably in 93% of cases, as hypoechoic, cystic space in the iris stroma which represents an enlarged iris vessel associated with the iris melanoma [3] (Fig. 6.4).

If the layering is distinct, the image is then frozen and a measurement vector is placed through the greatest depth on the screen image. The easiest method is to measure the total depth to the posterior iris surface. It is frequently impossible to tell exactly how much of the iris thickness is involved even in the presence of apparent layering.

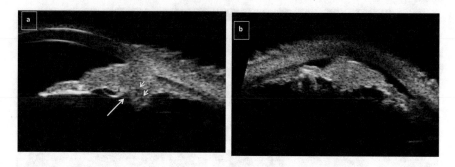

Fig. 6.4 Iris melanoma, **a** longitudinal scan showing an iris root mass invading the stroma and penetrating the posterior surface of iris pigment epithelium (long arrow) with evidence of hypoechoic cystic space denoting vascularity, **b** transverse scan of the iris melanoma showing its extension to the ciliary processes

6.1.2 Ciliary Body Tumors

UBM has been a valuable tool in the detection and management of small ciliary body tumors (less than 4 mm) [4]. It is of low to medium internal reflectivity. All ciliary body tumors must be followed circumferentially to assess their extent. Invasion of adjacent tissues may be evident, with a high-risk of extrascleral extension and metastasis [16, 17, 23, 36, 42] (Figs. 6.5, 6.6, 6.7 and 6.8).

Diffuse melanoma of the ciliary body with more than 180-degree involvement is called "ring melanoma". Ring melanomas often present atypically with glaucoma, retinal dialysis, or heterochromia

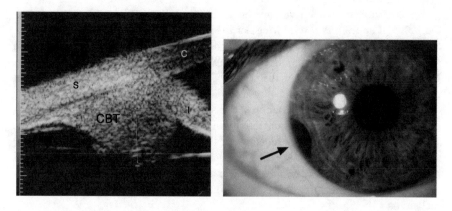

Fig. 6.5 Ultrasound biomicroscopy (UBM) of ciliary body tumor. (Top) UBM shows extension of the ciliary body tumor (CBT) into the iris. (S sclera; I iris; C cornea.) (Bottom)Clinical photograph of the same ciliary body tumor extending into the anterior chamber (arrow). (Weisbrod, Daniel J., et al. "Small ciliary body tumors: ultrasound biomicroscopic assessment and follow-up of 42 patients." American journal of ophthalmology) [4]

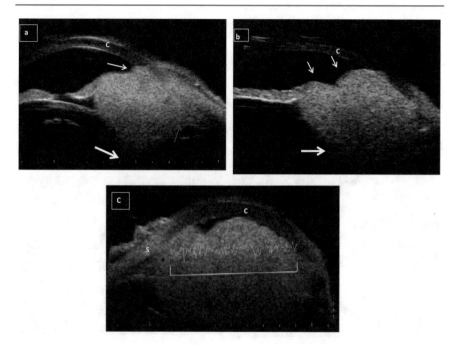

Fig. 6.6 A case of iridociliary melanoma **a** large iris tumor involving the iris root infiltrating the ciliary body (red arrow), with the anterior surface of the tumor reaching the cornea (thin arrow) obliterating the angle. **b** Lobulated tumor surface (thin arrows) with the tumor invading the posterior surface of the iris pigment epithelium and extending posteriorly (thick arrows in **a** and **b**). **c** Transverse UBM scan of the same tumor showing the lobulated surface of the tumor and the contact to the posterior corneal surface, with irregular internal reflectivity on the superimposed arbitrary A-scan. C: cornea S:sclera

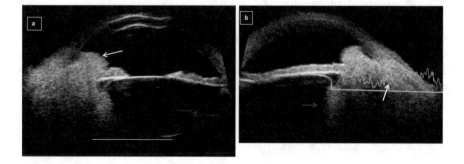

Fig. 6.7 Large iridociliary melanoma, **a** axial UBM scan demonstrating a mass infiltrating the iris root and extending anteriorly in the anterior chamber obliterating the angle and posteriorly almost reaching the lens capsule posteriorly (straight line). **b** Longitudinal scan showing infiltration of the ciliary body (white arrow) with the margin of the iridociliary tumor indenting the lens (red arrow). Note the irregular internal reflectivity on the superimposed arbitrary A-scan

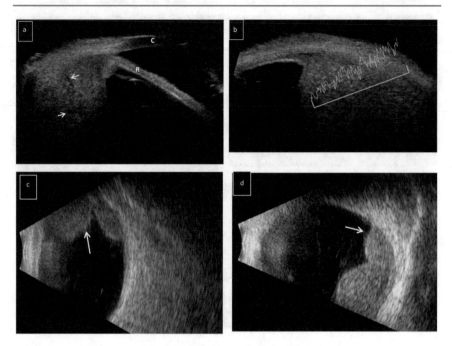

Fig. 6.8 Ciliochoroidal melanoma, **a** and **b** UBM of the ciliary body lesion extending posteriorly, however the posterior end is inaccessible by UBM. Note the cystic spaces(white arrows) **b** showing the superimposed A-scan with irregular internal reflectivity. **c** and **d** Longitudnal and Transverse B-Scan of the same patient showing the lobulated choroidal melanoma and its extension posteriorly (arrows)

6.2   Choroidal Melanoma

Choroidal melanoma is the most common primary intraocular tumor in adults, The diagnosis is based on clinical evaluation as well as several diagnostic techniques including ophthalmoscopy, ocular ultrasonography, fluorescein angiography and transillumination. The choroidal melanoma ultrasound has characteristic finding [19, 40, 44].

6.2.1   Shape and Reflectivity

Dome shaped or mushroom collar button configuration, as the tumor enlarges it can break through the Bruch's membrane giving rise to a mushroom or collar button shape. Choroidal melanoma is characterized by regular internal structure on B-scan and low to medium internal reflectivity on A-scan. Internal vascularity are traditionally seen as flickering spikes on the A scan; however, it disappears after treatment [18, 31].

6.2.2 Sound Attenuation

Sound attenuation is due to the densely homogeneous nature of the tumor. This is seen as decreased reflectivity at the tumor base on B-scan (acoustic hallowing) and a rapid decay of spikes on the A-scan, described as a steep angle kappa. Very dense tumors may also produce orbital shadowing.

6.2.3 Choroidal Excavation

This is an appearance produced by the contrast between the normal high reflective choroid surrounding the tumor and the low reflectivity of the densely homogenous tumor mass (the difference in reflectivity between the normal choroidal tissue and the abnormal tissue of the tumor replacing the choroid), which appear as curved appearance of the tumor base at its margin [5, 41].

6.2.4 Posterior Scleral Bowing

Posterior scleral bowing is caused by increased concavity of the sclera underlying the tumor seen near the tumor base as an area of low reflectivity, has been described in younger patients, and can be associated with scleral infiltration.

6.2.5 Exudative Retinal Detachment

Exudative retinal detachment indicates tumor activity, it often extends from the margins of the tumor and are also present in the lower periphery of the globe.

6.2.6 Extrascleral Extension

Extrascleral extension appears as one or more nodule adjacent to the base of the tumor, it must be 1.5 mm before it can be detected by ultrasound, where A-scan can assess the internal reflectivity and blood flow within the nodule. Diffuse melanoma can be difficult to diagnose, with high incidence of extrascleral extension [20, 47] (Figs. 6.9, 6.10, 6.11, 6.12, 6.13, 6.14, 6.15, 6.16, 6.17, 6.18, 6.19, 6.20 and 6.21).

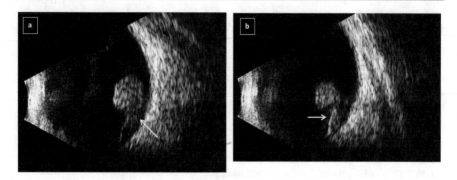

Fig. 6.9 Mushroom shaped choroidal melanoma, **a** transverse scan with decreased reflectivity at the base of the tumor, consistent with sound attenuation (white arrow) with the tumor showing the break in Bruch's membrane **b** transverse scan showing the periphery of the tumor showing the intact part of the Bruch's membrane

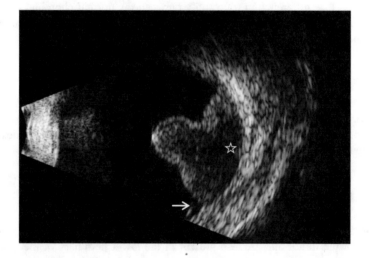

Fig. 6.10 Transverse scan of large collar button shaped choroidal melanoma with decreased reflectivity at the base of the tumor (star) consistent with sound attenuation, evidence of retinal detachment (white arrow)

N.B:

Vitreous and/or subretinal hemorrhage can rarely occur secondary to tumor growth

Irregular structure with high internal reflectivity are seen in very large tumors, suggesting hemorrhage and necrosis as well as dilated blood vessels.

Calcification may sometimes be seen on the surface.

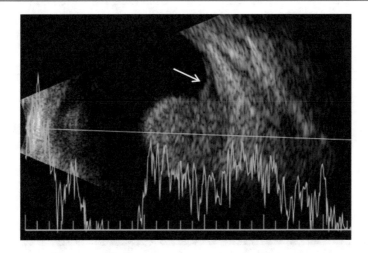

Fig. 6.11 Transverse scan of another patient showing Large Collar Button–shaped melanoma with irregular internal reflectivity in the superimposed A-scan, with secondary retinal detachment (white arrow)

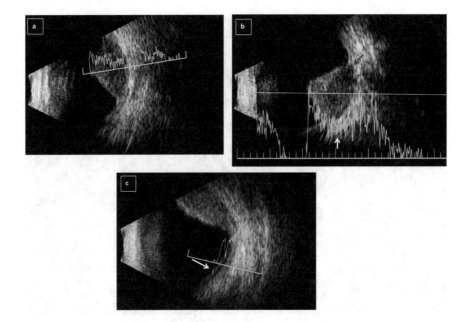

Fig. 6.12 a and **b** A large dome shaped choroidal melanoma with low internal reflectivity (white arrow), and a relatively echolucent base due to sound attenuation, **b** evidence of choroidal excavation due to curving of the tumour base at the margin of the tumour(red arrow), **c** showing shallow retinal detachment starting at the edge (white arrow)

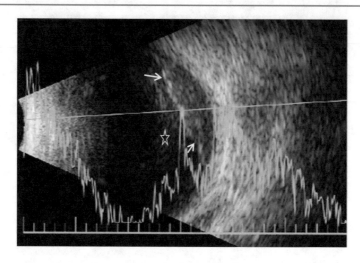

Fig. 6.13 Choroidal melanoma with irregular surface contour (white arrows) with low internal reflectivity in A-scan, vitreous hemorrhage (star), taking into consideration that the patient's main complaint was severe drop of vision

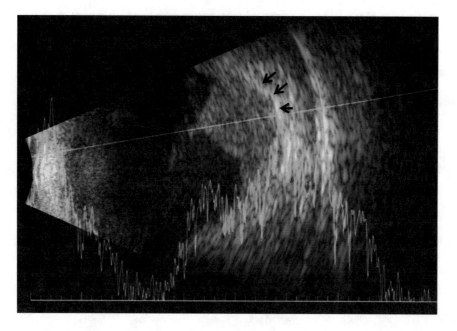

Fig. 6.14 Dome shaped melanoma with moderate internal reflectivity, with bowing of the sclera posterior to the tumor

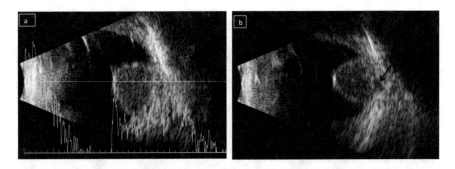

Fig. 6.15 a A Large dome shaped choroidal melanoma, with low internal reflectivity on A-scan, **b** evidence of extrascleral extension (black arrow)

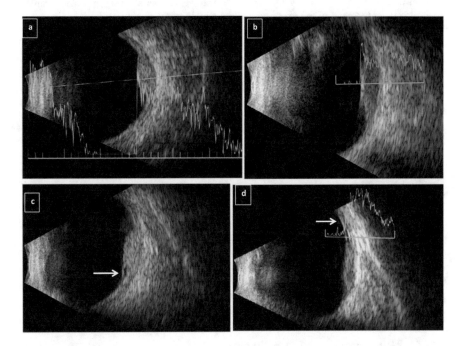

Fig. 6.16 Dome shaped choroidal melanoma, **a** and **b** showing the dome shaped mass with regular medium internal reflectivity on A-scan, **c** transverse scan showing retinal detachment at the tumor edge (white arrow) **d** longitudinal scan exposing the extend of the retinal detachment (white arrow)

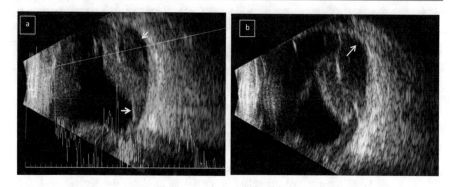

Fig. 6.17 a Longitudnal scan of Largre melanoma with low internal reflectivity, and an echolucent base due to sound attenuation at the base of the tumour(thin arrow), as well as retinal detachment at the margin (thick white arrow). **b** Transverse scan showing apparent choroidal excavation due to curving of the tumor base at the margin of the tumor (arrow)

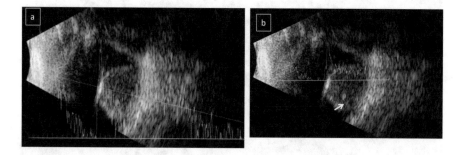

Fig. 6.18 a A Large dome shaped melanoma in the inferotemporal quadrant with low internal reflectivity on A-scan, **b** cystic space formation (white arrow)

Cystic spaces are not pathognomonic of choroidal melanoma, on the other hands large cystic cavities are more characteristic of ciliochoroidal melanoma.

6.2.7 Measurement of the Tumor

a) Tumor Height

* Longitudinal and transverse scan are used for accurate measurement of a lesion, axial and paraxial are suited for measuring lesions in the peripapillary lesions, peripheral lesions are better assessed with longitudinal scan.

* The lesion have to be centered in the echogram, and with adjusting the gain on medium gain setting, the inner sclera will be identified as the first distinct line at the

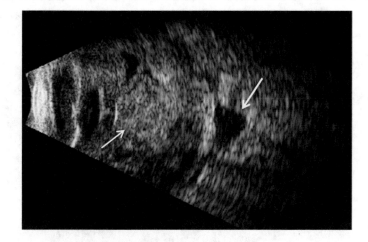

Fig. 6.19 Neglected large irregular shaped melanoma (thin arrow) filling the vitreous cavity, with extrascleral extension (white thick arrow) located near the optic disc

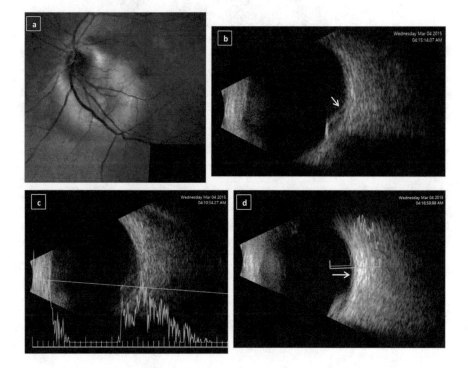

Fig. 6.20 Juxtapapillary malignant melanoma, **a** multicolored image of the tumor **b** a dome shaped mass with shallow retinal detachment (arrow) **c** showing the mass with low amplitude in A-san **d** note the extend of the shallow retinal detachment

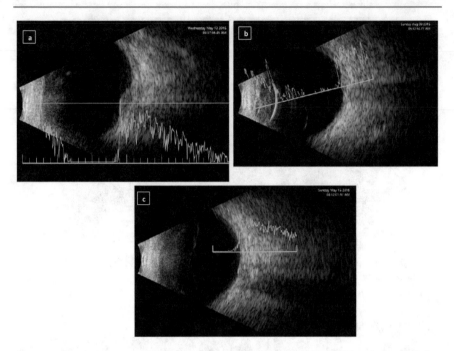

Fig. 6.21 Follow up of the same patient on Fig. 6.20 after receiving treatment, **a** 2 months after the first scan with increased echogenicity of the tumor and minimal decrease in the height of the tumor, **b** after 5 months of treatment note the decrease in size of the tumor and its high reflectivity on the superimposed A-scan, **c** disappearance of the mass and no evidence of retinal detachment after 14 months of treatment

base of the tumor. Once both the apex and inner sclera has been achieved, the height of the lesion can be measured using B and A-scan [26].

b) Tumor Base

The tumor base is measured by using both transverse and longitudinal scan, Transverse scan is used to measure the lateral diameter, whereas the longitudinal scan is used to measure the anteroposterior diameter [33] (Fig. 6.22).

c) Height-to-Base Ratio

The height-to-base ratio is calculated for each tumor. This ratio refers to the maximal prominence and the maximal base diameter of the tumor, In malignant melanoma there is a high height to base ratio [6, 41].

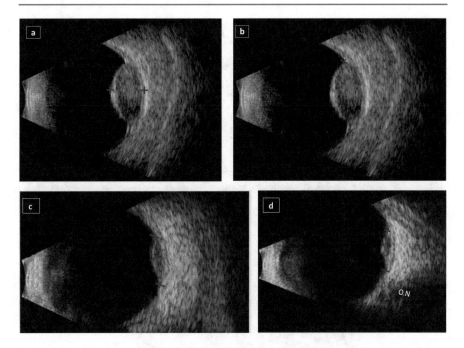

Fig. 6.22 Measurement of intraocular tumors: **a** Intraocular height measured by electronic cursors from the tumor surface to the inner sclera **b** Base measurement with placement of the cursors at the tumor margins - **c** Trasverse B-scan providing the lateral (circumferential) extent of the tumor **d** Longitudinal B-scan providing the anteroposterior extent of the tumor. (Optic nerve: O.N)

6.3 Choroidal Hemangioma

Choroidal hemangioma is a hamartomatous benign vascular tumor and considered to be congenital in origin. It is located in the peripapillary or the macular area [40, 46].

Choroidal hemangioma manifests in two subtypes: circumscribed or diffuse. Both subtypes can be bilateral and have no systemic associations.

6.3.1 Circumscribed Hemangioma

Dome shaped mass at the posterior pole with regular internal structure on B-scan and high internal reflectivity on A-scan [7, 24, 25]. There is no demonstrable internal blood flow, and serous retinal detachment can be present at tumor margins [37, 43] (Figs. 6.23 and 6.24).

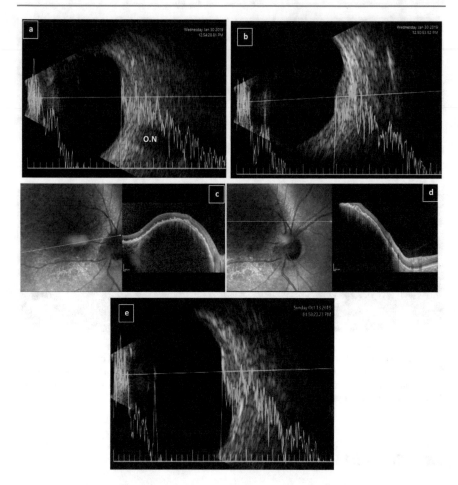

Fig. 6.23 a Longitudinal scan exposing a circumscribed hemangioma in the macular area, with moderate to high internal reflectivity on A-scan, **b** a transverse view of the tumor with regular internal reflectivity on A-scan, **c** and **d** enhanced depth imaging optical coherence tomography showing a hyporeflective dome shaped lesion with invisible overlying choriocapillaris and overlying mammillation of the outer layer. **e** Follow up after 9 months showing no signs of change in size or configuration (O.N: optic nerve)

6.3.2   Diffuse Hemangioma

In association with Sturge-Weber syndrome seen as a diffuse high reflective thickening of the posterior choroid that tapers off toward the equator [8]. The elevation in diffuse hemangiomas is not as high as in circumscribed lesions. Occasionally, areas of dome- shaped elevation may be seen within this diffuse area. Secondary retinal and choroidal detachment can occur in diffuse hemangiomas. Thickening of an adjacent extraocular muscle may also be observed [45].

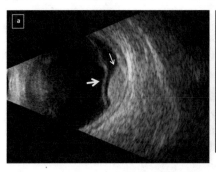
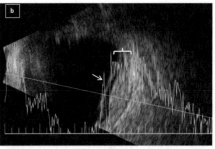

Fig. 6.24 **a** Transverse scan of a circumscribed hemangioma (thin arrow) with secondary retinal detachment (thick arrow), **b** superimposed A-scan of the tumor of regular moderate to high internal reflectivity (bracket). Note the high A-scan spike of the retina (thin arrow)

It is good to compare with the other eye, and look for the ipsilateral port-wine stain in an eye with unexplained unilateral choroidal thickening.

6.4 Metastsis

The choroid is the most common ophthalmic site for metastatic disease. Choroidal metastases can be either focal or multifocal with an irregular or bumpy surface contour with central excavation. A-scan will typically show moderate to high internal reflectivity with relatively irregular internal structures. No demonstrable internal blood flow. B-scan can identify mild to moderate elevation, as well as secondary exudative retinal detachment over the tumor surface. Vitreous and subretinal hemorrhage is rarely associated with metastatic carcinomas [34, 40] (Figs. 6.25, 6.26, 6.27 and 6.28).

Height-to-Base Ratio

Metastatic tumors had significantly lower height to base ratios than melanomas (p < 0.001).The metastases demonstrated height to base ratios ranging between 0.08 and 0.31 (mean 0.18 (SD 0.08)), whereas the height to base ratios of the melanomas ranged between 0.23 and 0.95 (mean 0.6 (SD 0.16) [6].

N.B

* Some metastatic tumors may exhibit a collar button shape which has been described, as seen in metastatic adenocarcinoma from the lung

* Another unusual finding is bullous choroidal detachments

* Low reflective internal echoes and presence of internal vascularity that may mimic a melanoma can be seen in metastatic 'oat cell carcinoma' of the lung.

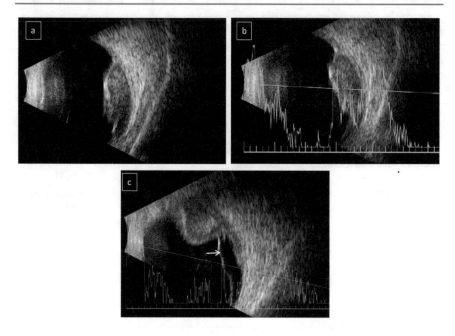

Fig. 6.25 a Highly elevated tumor with lobulated surface, **b** medium irregular reflectivity on A-scan, **c** secondary retinal detachment (white arrow)

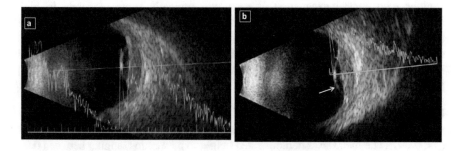

Fig. 6.26   Metastatic choroidal carcinoma of lung cancer, (**a** and **b**): transverse scans of a mildly elevated diffuse mass, associated with retinal detachment (white arrow) and irregular internal reflectivity in A-scan

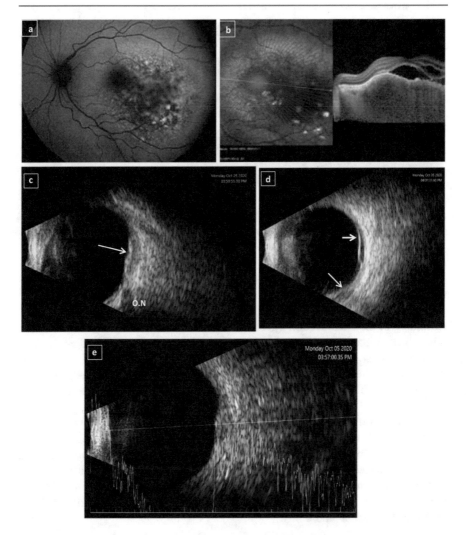

Fig. 6.27 **a** Metastatic choroidal carcinoma of breast cancer (**a**) autofluorescence of the tumor showing a lesion involving the macula with mottled hyperautofluorescence and hypoautofluorescence through the lesion course, **b** OCT showing hyporeflective choroidal mass with overlying irregular outer layers and subretinal fluid, **c** longitudinal B-scans showing the irregular surface of the tumor with moderate echogenicity, **d** transverse scan showing secondary retinal detachment (thick arrow) at the edge of the tumor(thin arrow), **e** moderate to high irregular internal reflectivity on A-scan

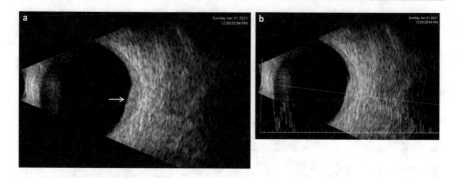

Fig. 6.28 Follow up of the same patient in Fig. 6.26 after 3 months of treatment by external beam irradiation, **a** the height of the tumor decreased from 2.9 to 2.1 mm and the base decreased from 10.4 to 8.8 mm **b** the superimposed A-scan of high irregular reflectivity

6.5 Choroidal Nevus

According to the classification system used in the Collaborative Ocular Melanoma Study, a choroidal nevus is a melanocytic choroidal lesion that is less than 5 mm in its largest basal diameter and smaller than 1 mm in its height [9, 10]. Thus, detection by echography might be difficult in some cases. B-scan of most elevated nevi appear with high reflectivity and nonvascular. It shows little or no growth on follow up.

Optical coherence tomography (OCT) and ultrasonography are important tools for the diagnosis of choroidal nevi. OCT can identify factors that increase the risk of malignant transformation, including subretinal fluid (even when the volume to be clinically detected is small), cystoid macular edema, and changes in the retinal pigment epithelium [11, 38]. Recently, enhanced depth imaging OCT (EDI-OCT) has been used in order to measure choroidal thickness in normal and pathologic eyes [12] (Figs. 6.29 and 6.30).

6.6 Choroidal Osteoma

Choroidal osteoma is a rare benign ossifying tumor of the choroid composed of mature calcified Bone, typically affecting healthy eyes of young females in the second and third decades.

It is typically a unilateral condition, presenting as a yellow-white to orange-red lesion in the juxtapapillary area. It produces very high internal reflectivity with orbital shadowing in ultrasound. A "Pseudo-optic nerve" or "double optic nerve" appearance may be seen [2, 21, 27–30, 35] (Figs. 6.31, 6.32 and 6.33).

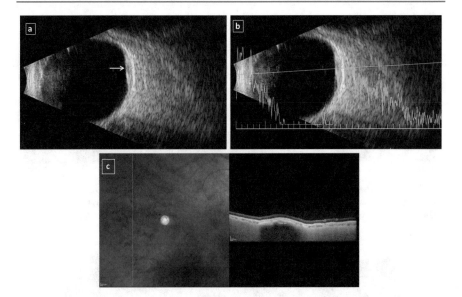

Fig. 6.29 Choroidal nevus, **a** longitudinal scan showing a mildly elevated lesion(arrow) **b** superimposed A-scan showing high internal reflectivity of the lesion **c** OCT of the lesion showing an elevated hyperreflective choroidal lesion with underlying shadowing compressing the overlying choriocapillaris with no evidence of intraretinal changes

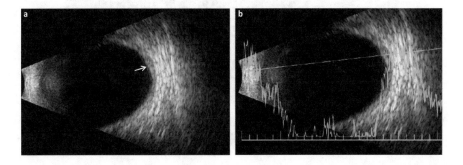

Fig. 6.30 Choroidal nevus, **a** transverse scan showing a small mildly elevated lesion **b** superimposed A-scan showing high internal reflectivity of the lesion

6.6.1   Sclerochoroidal Calcification

Sclerochoroidal calcification is a relatively rare condition characterized by yellow-white irregular subretinal lesions, usually presenting in the superotemporal mid-periphery of the fundus. The calcification is believed to be deposited at the sites of insertions of the oblique extraocular muscles in a similar way that Cogan scleral

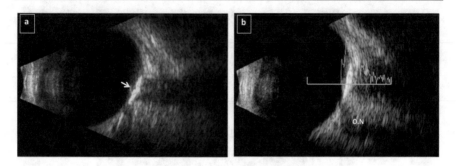

Fig. 6.31 **a** A case of osteoma with high echogenic lesion (white arrow) causing shadowing to the orbital tissue posteriorly, **b** longitudinal scan showing the osteoma in relation to the optic nerve "double optic nerve appearance" with high reflectivity of the osteoma on A-scan. Optic nerve: O.N

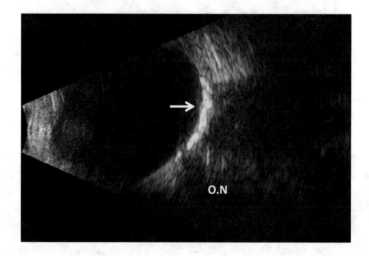

Fig. 6.32   A case of choroidal osteoma (short arrow) nasal to the optic disc with high echogenicity causing wide area of shadowing. Optic nerve: O.N

plaques are calcification at the insertions of the horizontal recti muscles. The pathology of calcification can be classified as dystrophic, metastatic, or idiopathic:

- Dystrophic processes involve normal calcium and phosphate metabolism with calcium salts deposition in abnormal tissue, such as in trauma or chronic inflammation [13, 32].
- Metastatic sclerochoroidal calcification (MSC) involve abnormal metabolism of calcium or phosphate, with resultant calcium salt deposition in normal tissues, occurring most commonly in primary hyperparathyroidism, pseudohypoparathyroidism, vitamin D intoxication, sarcoidosis, hypophosphatemia, and chronic renal failure [13].

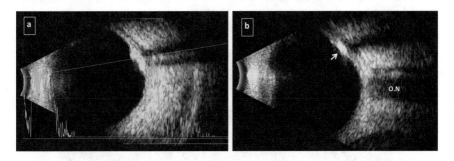

Fig. 6.33 a Transverse scan of osteoma of irregular surface with high echogenicity causing shadowing "pseudo-optic nerve appearance" with high reflectivity on A-scan, **b** longitudinal scan showing the osteoma (short arrow) in relation to the optic nerve (O.N)

– Sclerochoroidal calcification is considered idiopathic when metastatic and dystrophic causes have been ruled out, calcium and phosphate metabolism is normal, and calcium salt deposition occurs in normal tissue [14]. Idiopathic sclerochoroidal calcification is a lesion of calcium salt precipitation in the sclera and choroid, often discovered asymptomatically on routine examination with normal visual acuity and visual fields [48] (Figs. 6.34 and 6.35).

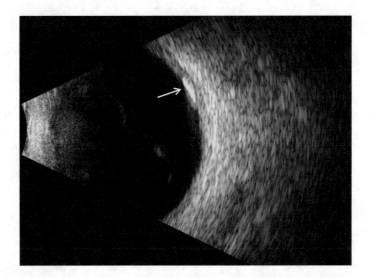

Fig. 6.34 Idiopathic sclerochoroidal calcification in the superotemporal quadrant, with high echogenicity

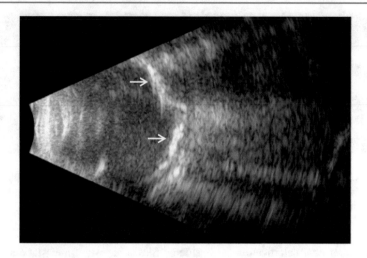

Fig. 6.35 A case with an old history of trauma showing multiple sclerochoroidal calcified plaques of high reflectivity, causing shadowing to the orbital tissue posteriorly

Table for differential diagnosis of the most common introcular lesions:

Type	Shape	Ultrasound features
Malignant choroidal melanoma	Collar button or dome-shape appearance	– Regular internal structure – Low to moderate internal reflectivity – Acoustic hollowness – Choroidal excavation – Internal vascularity
Choroidal Metastasis	Diffuse, lobulated, irregular or multifocal lesion present at posterior pole	– Irregular or regular internal structure – Medium to high internal reflectivity – Nonvascular
Choroidal Hemangioma	Dome-shaped, diffuse in Sturge-Weber syndrome	– Regular internal structure – High internal reflectivity
Choroidal nevus	Dome-shaped, flat or minimally elevated lesion, less than 2 mm in size	– Medium to high internal reflectivity – Nonvascular – Minimal or no growth
Choroidal Osteoma	Plaque-like lesion	– High reflectivity, even at low gain – May cause posterior shadowing

References

1. Pavlin CJ, Stuart Foster F. Ultrasound biomicroscopy of the eye. Springer Science & Business Media; 2012.
2. Bhende M, et al. Atlas of ophthalmic ultrasound and ultrasound biomicroscopy. JP Medical Ltd; 2013.
3. Elkady S. Ultrasound biomicroscopy: role in diagnosis of iris and ciliary body tumours. Med J Cairo Univ. 2011;79.2.
4. Weisbrod DJ, et al. Small ciliary body tumors: ultrasound biomicroscopic assessment and follow-up of 42 patients. Am J Ophthalmol. 2006;141(4):622–8.
5. Byrne SF. Ultrasound of the eye and orbit. Mosby Incorporated; 2002.
6. Sobottka B, et al. Choroidal metastases and choroidal melanomas: comparison of ultrasonographic findings. Br J Ophthalmol. 1998;82(2):159–61.
7. Soucek P, Cihelková I. Evaluation of subretinal fluid absorption by optical coherence tomography in circumscribed choroidal hemangioma after photodynamic therapy with Verteporfin. Neuroendocrinol Lett. 2004;25(1/2):109–14.
8. Spraul, CW, et al. Mushroom-shaped choroidal hemangioma. Am J Ophthalmol. 1996;122 (3):434–6.
9. Collaborative Ocular Melanoma Study Group Factors predictive of growth and treatment of small choroidal melanoma: COMS report no. 5. Arch Ophthalmol. 1997;115:1537–44.
10. Jonas JB, et al. Choroidal nevi in adult Chinese. Ophthalmology. 2008;115(6):1102.
11. Martins MF, et al. Comparisons of choroidal nevus measurements obtained using 10-and 20-MHz ultrasound and spectral domain optical coherence tomography. Arquivos brasileiros de oftalmologia. 2017;80(2):78–83.
12. Basdekidou C, et al. Flat choroidal nevus inaccessible to ultrasound sonography evaluated by enhanced depth imaging optical coherence tomography. Case Rep Ophthalmol. 2011;2 (2):185–8.
13. Honavar SG, et al. Sclerochoroidal calcification: clinical manifestations and systemic associations. Arch Ophthalmol. 2001;119(6):833–40.
14. Kim M, Pian D, Ferrucci S. Idiopathic sclerochoroidal calcification. Optom-J Am Optom Assoc. 2004;75(8):487–95.
15. Mithal KN, et al. Role of echography in diagnostic dilemma in choroidal masses. Indian J Ophthalmol. 2014;62(2):167.
16. Conway RM, et al. Ultrasound biomicroscopy: role in diagnosis and management in 130 consecutive patients evaluated for anterior segment tumours. Br J Ophthalmol. 2005;89 (8):950–5.
17. Bianciotto C, et al. Assessment of anterior segment tumors with ultrasound biomicroscopy versus anterior segment optical coherence tomography in 200 cases. Ophthalmology. 2011;118(7):1297–302.
18. Wang T-J, et al. Characteristic ultrasonographic findings of choroidal tumors. J Med Ultrasound. 2003;11(2):55–9.
19. Peyster RG, et al. Choroidal melanoma: comparison of CT, fundoscopy, and US. Radiology. 1985;156(3):675–80.
20. Shultz RW, Ahuja Y, Pulido JS. Bidirectional thermotherapy for choroidal melanoma. Eye. 2011;25(8):1094.
21. Lehto KS, Tommila PV, Karma A. Choroidal osteoma: clues to diagnosis. Acta Ophthalmol Scand. 2007;85(2):218–20.
22. Gentile RC, et al. Ciliary body enlargement and cyst formation in uveitis. Br J Ophthalmol. 1996;80(10):895–9.

23. Shields JA, et al. Ciliochoroidal nerve sheath tumor simulating a malignant melanoma. Retina. 1997;17(5):459–60.
24. Khuu T, Hoffman DJ. Circumscribed choroidal hemangioma: A case report and review of the literature. Optom-J Am Optom Assoc. 2006;77(8):384–91.
25. Arevalo JF, et al. Circumscribed choroidal hemangioma: characteristic features with indocyanine green videoangiography. Ophthalmology. 2000;107(2):344–50.
26. Russo A, et al. Diffusion-weighted magnetic resonance imaging and ultrasound evaluation of choroidal melanomas after proton-beam therapy. La Radiol Med. 2015;120(7):634–40.
27. Empeslidis T, et al. Diagnosis and monitoring of choroidal osteoma through multimodal imaging. Case Rep Med. 2014;2014.
28. Dinah C, Sandinha T. Enhanced depth imaging as an adjunctive tool in the diagnosis of decalcified choroidal osteoma. Eye. 2014;28(3):356–8.
29. Navajas EV, et al. Multimodal fundus imaging in choroidal osteoma. Am J Ophthalmol. 2012;153(5):890–5.
30. Abramson DH, et al. Choroidal osteoma: acoustic shadowing and reduplication echoes. Insight- J Am Soc Ophthalmic Regist Nurses. 1996;21(4):118–9.
31. Fuller DG, et al. Ultrasonographic features of choroidal malignant melanomas. Arch Ophthalmol. 1979;97(8):1465–72.
32. Wong CM, Kawasaki BS. Idiopathic sclerochoroidal calcification. Optom Vis Sci. 2014;91 (2):e32–7.
33. Marchini G, Tosi R, Ghimenton C. Measurement of tumour height and base diameter in choroidal melanoma. Comparison between ultrasonography and histology. In: Ultrasonography in ophthalmology XV. Springer, Dordrecht; 1997. pp. 93–100.
34. Mahajan A, et al. Ocular neoplastic disease. In: Seminars in ultrasound, CT and MRI, vol. 32, no. 1. WB Saunders; 2011.
35. Shields CL, et al. Regression of extrafoveal choroidal osteoma following photodynamic therapy. Arch Ophthalmol. 2008;126(1):135–7.
36. Vallejo-Vicente E, et al. Pigmented tumor of the ciliary body: benign or malignant ? Arch Span Soc Ophthalmol. 2013;88(12):485–8.
37. Irvine F, et al. Retinal vasoproliferative tumors: surgical management and histological findings. Arch Ophthalmol. 2000;118(4):563–9.
38. Shields JA, et al. The differential diagnosis of posterior uveal melanoma. Ophthalmology. 1980;87(6):518–22.
39. Gündüz K, et al. The use of ultrasound biomicroscopy in the evaluation of anterior segment tumors and simulating conditions. Ophthalmologica. 2007;221.5:305–12.
40. Coleman DJ, et al. Ultrasonic diagnosis of tumors of the choroid. Arch Ophthalmol. 1974;91 (5): 344–54.
41. Sobottka B, Kreissig I. Ultrasonography of metastases and melanomas of the choroid. Curr Opin Ophthalmol. 1999;10(3):164–7.
42. Kawana K, et al. Ultrasound biomicroscopic findings of ciliary body malignant melanoma. Jpn J Ophthalmol. 2004;48(4):412–4.
43. Piñeiro-Ces A, et al. Diagnóstico ecográfico de los tumores vasoproliferativos del fondo de ojo. Arch Soc Esp Oftalmol. 2011;86:247–53.
44. Chaudhari H, et al. Role of ultrasonography in evaluation of orbital lesions. Trauma. 2013;20:20.
45. Singh AD, Lorek BH. Ophthalmic ultrasonography e-book: expert consult-online and print. Elsevier Health Sciences; 2011.
46. Rojanaporn D, Kaliki S, Ferenczy SR, Shields CL. Enhanced depth imaging optical coherence tomography of circumscribed choroidal hemangioma in 10 consecutive cases. Middle East Afr J Ophthalmol. 2015;22(2):192–7. https://doi.org/10.4103/0974-9233.150629.

47. Jacobsen BH, Ricks C, Harrie RP. Ocular ultrasound versus MRI in the detection of extrascleral extension in a patient with choroidal melanoma. BMC Ophthalmol. (2018);18(1).
48. Sivalingam A, et al. Idiopathic sclerochoroidal calcification. Ophthalmology. 1991;98 (5):720–4.

Inflammatory Diseases of the Eye

7

7.1 Anterior Uveitis

There are numerous causes of anterior uveitis including sarcoidosis [1], Reiter's disease, inflammatory bowel disease, juvenile idiopathic arthritis and infectious condition as herpes simplex and varicella-zoster virus. The clinical presentation of acute anterior uveitis is sudden onset of pain, photophobia & redness. Anterior uveitis also includes iritis, iridocyclitis.

*Ultrasound biomicroscopy features include

(A) Numerous cells in the anterior and posterior chamber (Fig. 7.1).
(B) Partial angle closure by the formation of peripheral anterior synechiae (PAS). With progression of PAS, the intraocular pressure gradually increases, especially if the ciliary body is still functioning (Fig. 7.2).
(C) Posterior synechiae, Iris bombe and irideocorneal touch.
(D) Iris atrophy and iris nodule [2, 3] (Fig. 7.3).
(E) Striking edema in the iris and ciliary body, as well as a variety of exudates (massive, linear, dotted or with irregular shapes) adjacent to these affected tissues and in the anterior vitreous at the peak of the inflammation [4–6] (Fig. 7.4).
(F) Ciliary body granuloma [7, 8] (Fig. 7.5).

© The Author(s), under exclusive license to Springer Nature Switzerland AG 2021   181
R. Abbas, *Ophthalmic Ultrasonography and Ultrasound Biomicroscopy*,
https://doi.org/10.1007/978-3-030-76979-6_7

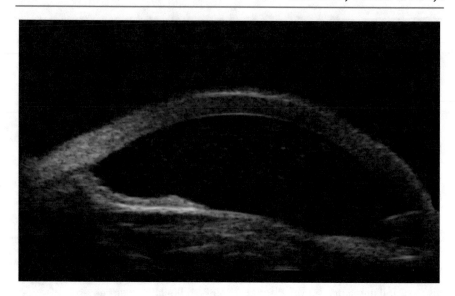

Fig. 7.1 Axial UBM scan showing multiple echoes in the anterior chamber (dots-like) consistent with inflammatory cells

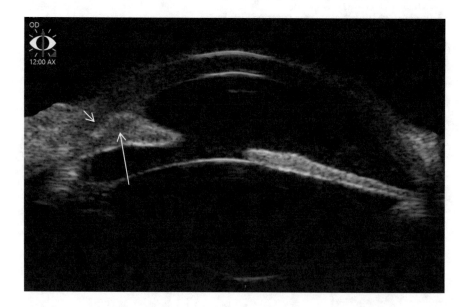

Fig. 7.2 Axial UBM scan showing the superior and inferior quadrant, with multiple echoes filling the anterior chamber (inflammatory cells). Evidence of iris granuloma with hypoechoic center (white long arrow) and intact iris pigment epithelium. Note the anterior synechiae in the inferior quadrant at 6 o'clock (white short arrow)

Fig. 7.3 Tuberculosis iris granuloma (**a**) Longitudinal scan showing iris granuloma with intact iris pigment epithelium, (**b**) transverse UBM scan exposing the granuloma with hypoechoic center and intact iris pigment epithelium

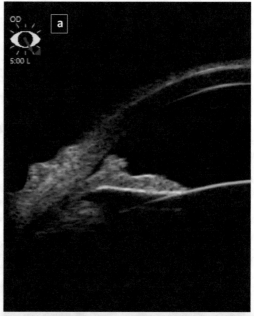

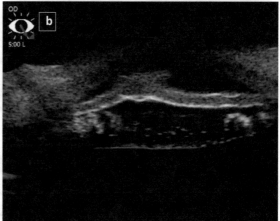

7.2 Intermediate Uveitis

*Intermediate uveitis is an intraocular inflammation involving primarily the anterior vitreous, peripheral retina and pars plana.

*The etiology may be idiopathic, however, there are several associated diseases such as multiple sclerosis, optic neuritis, autoimmune corneal endotheliopathy, sarcoidosis, thyroid diseases and inflammatory bowel diseases. Furthermore, a

Fig. 7.4 a Longitudinal UBM scan demonstrating dense inflammatory cells in the anterior chamber, with peripheral anterior synechiae (white arrow). **b** Longitudinal UBM scan showing inflammatory membranes around the ciliary body extending to the pars plana (red arrow) and surrounding the zonules (white arrow), **c** transverse UBM scan showing ciliary body processes infiltrated by inflammatory membranes (white arrow)

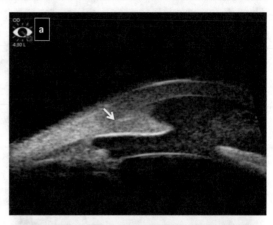

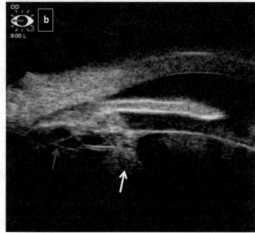

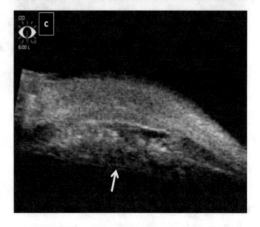

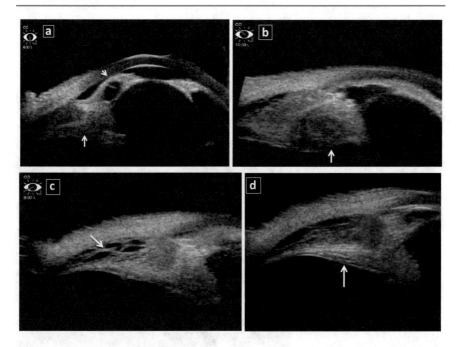

Fig. 7.5 a Axial UBM scan demonstrating occlusio pupillea causing iris bombe and iridocorneal touch (short arrow) with an inflammatory membrane around the ciliary body (long arrow). Note the enlargement of the ciliary body denoting ciliary body edema. **b** A granuloma of the ciliary body (white arrow). **c** Longitudinal scan exposing the ciliary body effusion, **d** Longitudinal UBM scan showing the inflammatory membranes extending from the ciliary body to the pars plana (white arrow)

number of infectious agents have been associated with the syndrome including Borrelia burgdorferi (Lyme disease), Toxocara canis (Toxocariasis), Whipple's bacilli (Whipple's disease), Epstein-Barr virus, HTLV I and HIV.

*Symptoms include blurry vision, floaters and distortion of central vision. The syndrome is traditionally bilateral in 80% of the patients and chronic with periods of exacerbation and remission. Clinical presentation includes mild to moderate anterior chamber inflammation, thin keratic precipitates in the inferior portion of the cornea, autoimmune endotheliopathy, vitritis, vasculitis in the peripheral retina, intravitreal "*snowballs*," retinal "*snowbanking*," optic neuritis and cystoid macular edema [9–11].

Pars planitis is an idiopathic intermediate uveitis characterized by chronic inflammatory deposits (snowbanks) in the area of the pars plana, and vitreous cells, which can also appear clumped together as "snowballs", and it is typically bilateral.

Fig. 7.6 **a** Longitudinal
UBM scan showing dense
inflammatory membrane
(double arrow)around the
ciliary body extending to pars
plana and covering the
zonules reaching to the lens
equator (white arrow),
b transverse scan showing the
membranes hiding the ciliary
processes

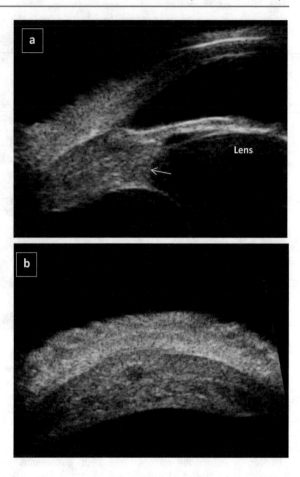

UBM Features

(A) Exudative material or membranes over the pars plana and peripheral retina mostly inferiorly [12] (Fig. 7.6).

(B) A low reflective mass over the pars plana and ciliary body region suggestive of exudates, along with low reflective ciliary body thickening suggestive of ciliary body edema as a sign of active pars planitis [13, 14] (Fig. 7.5).

(C) Chronic stages show high reflective pars plana membranes all around or in a few quadrants with or without traction on the ciliary body and peripheral retina.

(D) Ciliary process atrophy with subsequent hypotony is an important prognostic tool before cataract surgery.

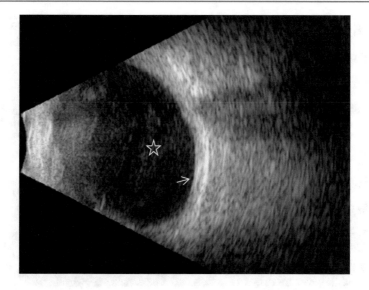

Fig. 7.7 Axial B-scan of the same patient showing echoes filling the vitreous cavity denoting vitritis (star) and retinochoroidal thickening (white arrow)

7.3 Posterior Uveitis

*Posterior uveitis may occur as idiopathic or as part of autoimmune diseases affecting body systems such as sarcoidosis, collagen vascular disorders, White dot syndrome. It may also occur with infectious underlying cause as TB, viral posterior uveitis, fungal, syphilis and toxoplasmosis. Primary site of inflammation can be the choroid, retina or both with variable involvement of the vitreous.

The ultrasound findings most commonly seen in posterior uveitis include vitritis [15], posterior vitreous detachment (PVD), subvitreal opacity, retinochoroidal thickening, macular oedema, Choroidal thickening which can be localized or diffuse, and choroidal detachment. Longstanding uveitis can lead to formation of cataract and cyclitic membrane [16] (Figs. 7.7, 7.8, 7.9, 7.10, and 7.11).

7.4 Endophthalmitis

There are no clear diagnostic criteria for infectious endophthalmitis. The diagnosis is suspected clinically when cardinal signs of inflammation are present, including conjunctival injection, pain, hypopyon, and decreased vision. Endophthalmitis is a potentially devastating intraocular inflammation occurring as a complication of intraocular surgery, trauma, systemic infection or uveitis [17].

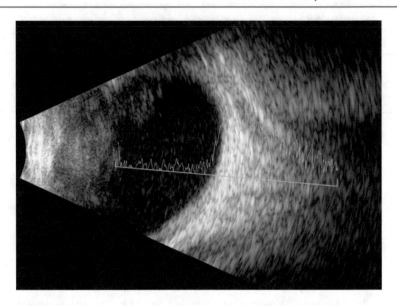

Fig. 7.8 Transverse scan showing echoes almost filling the vitreous cavity of low reflectivity in the superimposed arbitrary A-scan, denoting vitritis

On B-scan ultrasonography, the vitreous involvement is characterized by numerous low-amplitude mobile echoes in the vitreous. Membranes appear as fine dots and lines of varying densities [18, 19]. Presence of thicker echoes anteriorly suggests an anterior locus of infection. Some patients demonstrated large vitreous vacuoles with thickening of the vacuolar wall and vitreous opacities also known as cobweb-shaped membranes. A-scan of moderately severe endophthalmitis produces a chain of low amplitude spikes within the vitreous cavity. In posterior vitreous detachment, echoes in the subvitreal space suggests active inflammation [20, 21] (Figs. 7.12, 7.13 and 7.14).

Other common ultrasonographic findings include choroidal thickening, retinochoroidal thickening, choroidal and/or retinal detachment and optic nerve edema [22] (Figs. 7.15, 7.16, 7.17, and 7.18).

7.5 Vogt-Koyanagi-Harada

Vogt-Koyanagi-Harada disease is a cell-mediated autoimmune disorder involving melanocyte containing organs, including uvea, skin, inner ears, and choroid plexus [23]. It is an idiopathic bilateral,chronic granulomatous panuveitis, associated with exudative retinal detachment and with neurological, auditory and integumentary manifestations [24].

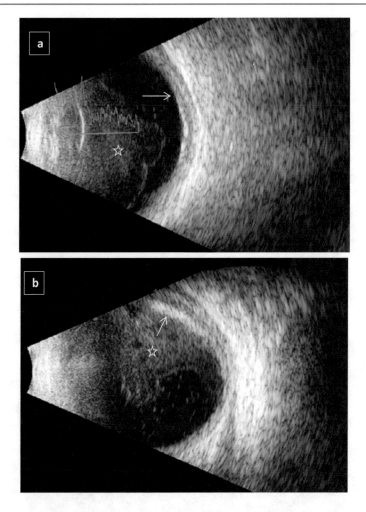

Fig. 7.9 A case of posterior uveitis, (**a**) echoes of low reflectivity collapsed anteriorly (vitritis) (star in **a** and **b**) with posterior hyaloid detachment and retinochoroidal thickening (arrow) (**b**) longitudinal B-scan exposing the ciliochoroidal detachment anteriorly (arrow)

VKH disease may be divided into two stages:

*Acute onset VKH, characterized by severe sub-retinal fluid accumulation with occasional exudative retinal detachment extending to the peripheral retina and extending anteriorly to cause bullous detachment. Additionally, it is characterized by diffuse severe choroidal thickening, as well as variable degrees of vitritis [25, 26].

*Chronic recurrent VKH includes several clinical features such as choroidal thickening and variable vitritis with occasional subretinal fluid accumulation and a recurrent granulomatous anterior uveitis.

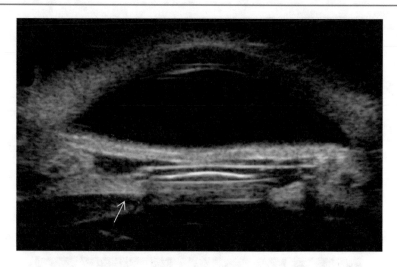

Fig. 7.10 Axial UBM scan showing IOL with cyclitic membrane posteriorly (white arrow) representing longstanding uveitis

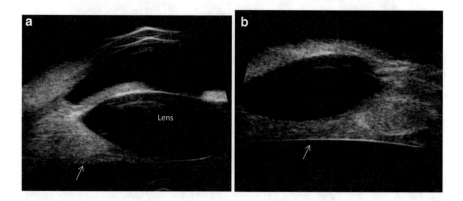

Fig. 7.11 a Longitudinal UBM scan showing a thick membrane extending from ciliary body reaching the lens equator to the posterior capsule, **b** axial scan exploring the extension of the membrane to the opposite side (consistent with cyclitic membrane)

Ultrasonography Findings of VKH

Echographic findings in VKH include diffuse, low to medium reflective thickening of the choroid posteriorly, which typically pronounced in the peripapillary region, serous retinal detachment, located inferiorly or in the posterior pole, mild vitreous opacities with no posterior vitreous detachment (Figs. 7.19, 7.20).

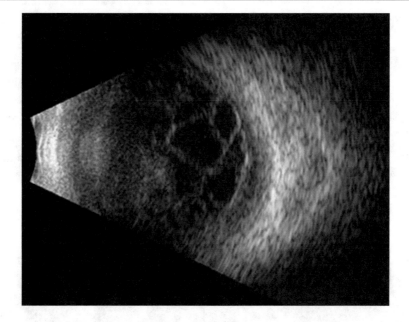

Fig. 7.12 A case of endophthalmitis after penetrating trauma showing multiple vitreous membranes with a Cobweb appearance

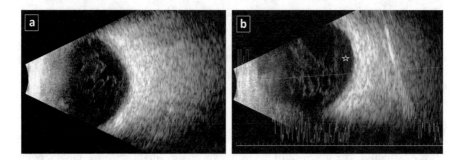

Fig. 7.13 A case of endophthalmitis, **a** multiple echoes and membranes forming the cobweb appearance, **b** transverse scan of another quadrant showing multiple echoes in the subvitreal space (star) denoting active inflammation

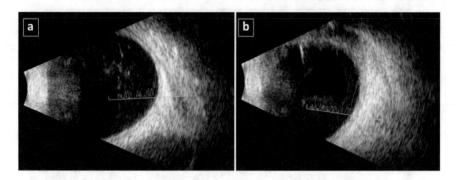

Fig. 7.14 A case of active endophthalmitis, **a** and **b** longitudinal and transverse B-scan showing multiple echoes in the subvitreal space with low reflectivity on the superimposed A-scan

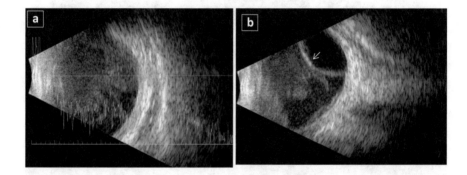

Fig. 7.15 A case of endophthalmitis, **a** transverse B-scan showing multiple echoes and membranes of low to moderate echogenicity filling the vitreous cavity with irregular internal reflectivity in A-scan **b** longitudinal B-scan exposing a bullous choroidal detachment at one quadrant (white arrow)

*UBM may demonstrate

Shallow anterior chambers during the active phase, angle closure, ciliary body thickening, decreased internal echo reflection of the ciliary body stroma, obscured appearance of the ciliary processes, supraciliary effusion and ciliochoroidal detachment in certain cases [23] (Fig. 7.21).

7.6 Toxocariasis

*Ocular toxocariasis is an infection caused by roundworms. Ocular toxocariasis is generally unilateral disease and during childhood can results in unilateral loss of vision [27]. Toxocariesis may present clinically as a lesion in the posterior or

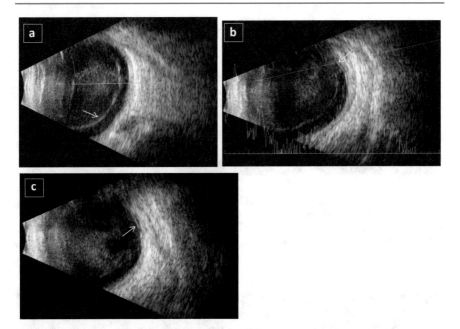

Fig. 7.16 A case of endophthalmitis, **a** multiple echoes of moderate amplitude with evidence of thickened PVD (white arrow), **b** shallow localized tractional retinal detachment caused by the adherent inflammatory membranes and the posterior hyaloid **c** longitudinal scan with low gain to reveal the localized shallow retinal detachment (white arrow)

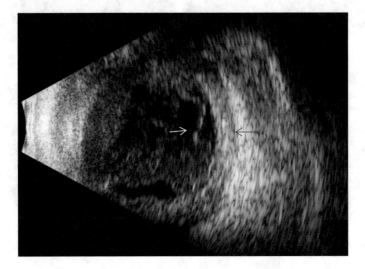

Fig. 7.17 A case of endophthalmitis: transverse B-scan showing dense echoes and membranes filling most of the vitreous cavity with evidence of retinal detachment (white arrow) with choroid and scleral thickening and mild widening with inflammation of the sub-Tenon's space (red arrow)

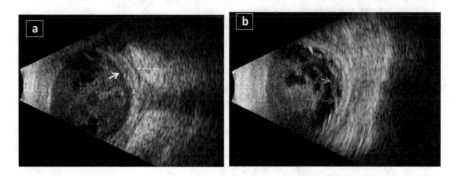

Fig. 7.18 A case of endophthalmitis, **a** axial B-scan showing dense echoes and membranes filling the vitreous cavity with retinochoroidal and scleral thickening (thick white arrow) and widening with inflammation of the sub-Tenon's space (thin white arrow), **b** transverse B-scan of multiple focal traction retinal detachment (red arrows) caused by inflammatory membranes (white arrow)

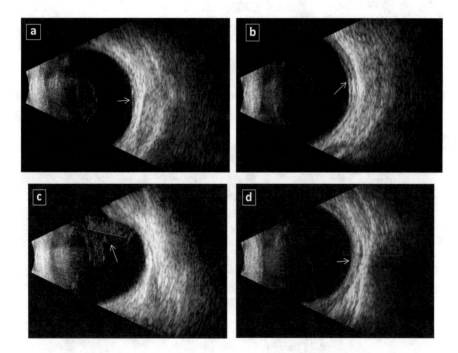

Fig. 7.19 A case of VKH, **a** and **b** shallow exudative detachment (arrow) **c** multiple echoes of low amplitude in the anterior vitreous cavity (vitritis) **d** choroidal and scleral thickening (arrow)

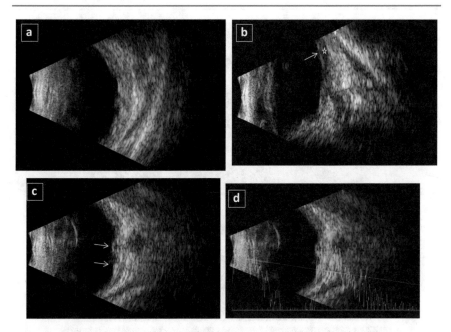

Fig. 7.20 A case of VKH, **a** and **c** showing shallow irregular exudative retinal detachment (arrows) in the posterior pole, (**b**) longitudinal scan showing the extend of the retinal detachment (arrow) and the subretinal fluid (star), **d** thickened choroid and decreased reflectivity of the choroid with low to medium reflectivity in A-scan (red arrow)

peripheral retina. Granulomas tend to appear in the inferonasal region. Detachment of the ciliary body or choroid usually occurs in the attachment region of granulomas.

UBM in Peripheral granulomas is manifested as hyperechoic solid masses with rough borders, of which the majority located on the surface of the ciliary body or peripheral choroid featuring tight adhesion but clear boundary with the ciliary body [28].

Thick vitreous strands could be found on the surface of the granulomas or the adjacent orbital tissue.Other peripheral lesions include vitreous strands, peripheral traction retinal detachment and tractional cyclodialysis.

UBM and ultrasonography reveal similar pseudocystic changes in the peripheral vitreous that seem to put tractional forces on the peripheral retina [29] (Fig. 7.22).

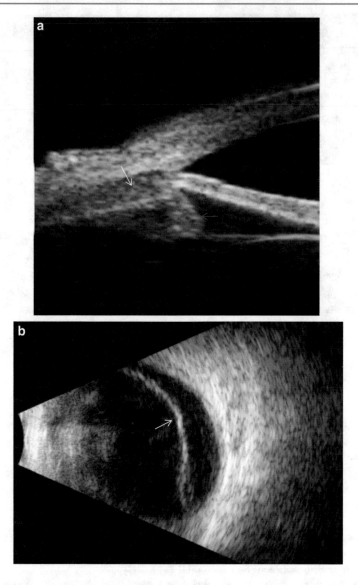

Fig. 7.21 A case of VKH: **a** UBM showing the ciliary body surrounded with inflammatory membranes (red arrow) with ciliary body oedema and low echogenicity of the ciliary body stroma (white arrow), **b** B-scan showing exudative retinal detachment (white arrow)

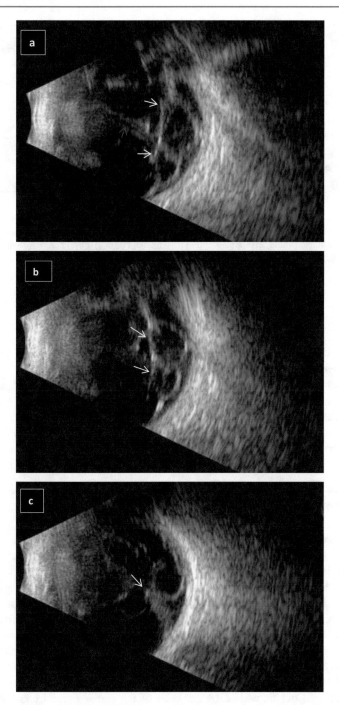

Fig. 7.22 A case of toxocariasis, **a** and **b** multiple vitreous membranes (red arrow) extending from the retrolenticular area forming a pseudocystic changes in the peripheral vitreous (white arrows) causing traction retinal detachment (arrow in **c**)

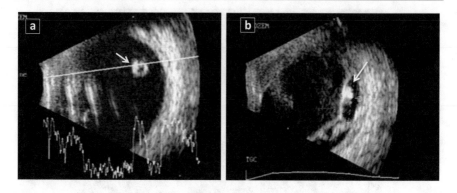

Fig. 7.23 a B-scan ultrasonography showing intravitreal cyst with scolex (white arrow), **b** showing subretinal cyst (red arrow) with scolex (white arrow), (Ganesh, Sudha K., and Priyanka, Analysis of clinical profile, investigation, and management of ocular cysticercosis seen at a tertiary referral centre) [35]

7.7 Cysticercosis

Cysticercosis is caused by *Cysticercus cellulosae*, the larval form of pork tapeworm, *Taenia solium.*

Cysticercosis has a characteristic echographic appearance, a well outlined round to oval echolucent cyst with an echo dense nodule adjacent to the inner wall of the cyst representing the scolex. The scolex exhibits spontaneous movements on kinetic scan. Extensive vitreous echoes, membranes and retinal detachment can develop in response to inflammation caused by the dead cyst [30–34] (Figs. 7.23 and 7.24).

7.8 Lens and IOL Induced Uveitis

Lens induced uveitis is an inflammatory response to lens matter release into the vitreous cavity. It typically develops after traumatic or surgical perforation of the lens capsule, or in some cases of hypermature cataract.

Untreated hypermature cataract can result in leakage of the lens material into the anterior chamber which could develop into phacolytic glaucoma or phacoanaphylactic uveitis. In retained lens matter or lens fragment in the vitreous cavity, the lens matter are surrounded by inflammatory vitreous opacities and membrane which is well seen by ultrasound. Management and surgical plan entirely dependent on the ultrasound and UBM findings as dispersed lens matter completely precludes clinical examination (Figs. 7.25 and 7.26).

IOL induced uveitis caused by irritation of the ocular tissue by an intraocular lens where a combination of uveitis, glaucoma and hyphema can occur due to frequent chafing of the iris and ciliary body by the IOL haptics [37]. UBM can

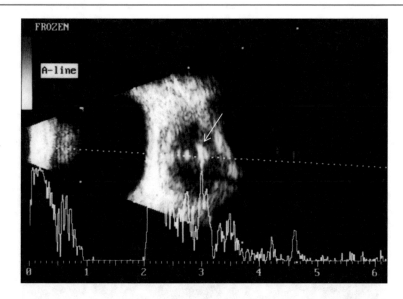

Fig. 7.24 Ultrasound A and B scan of the orbit showing a retrobulbar cyst with scolex (white arrow). (Pushker, N., Bajaj, M.S. and Betharia, S.M. (2002), Orbital and adnexal cysticercosis. Clinical & Experimental Ophthalmology) [36]

predict the relationship of the IOL haptic to the iris and angle structures, as well as retained lens matter within the capsular bag [38] and other associated findings may include ciliary body edema, peripheral anterior synechiae and cyclitic membranes (Figs. 7.27, 7.28, and 7.29).

7.9 Scleritis

Scleritis is a severe, destructive, vision-threatening inflammation involving the deep episclera and sclera. It can be diffuse, nodular or necrotizing. It can either affect the anterior or posterior aspect of the eye.

Anterior scleritis, which is more common, may be diffuse, nodular, or necrotizing [39]. Posterior scleritis is described as involvement of the sclera posterior to the insertion of the recti muscles.. The etiology is commonly idiopathic, however, up to 50% of scleritis have evidence of an underlying connective tissue disease or infectious etiology.

Episcleritis is usually a diffuse process or less commonly a nodular form of episcleral inflammation. It appears in UBM as episcleral thickening with low to medium reflectivity without involvement of the scleral tissue (Fig. 7.30).

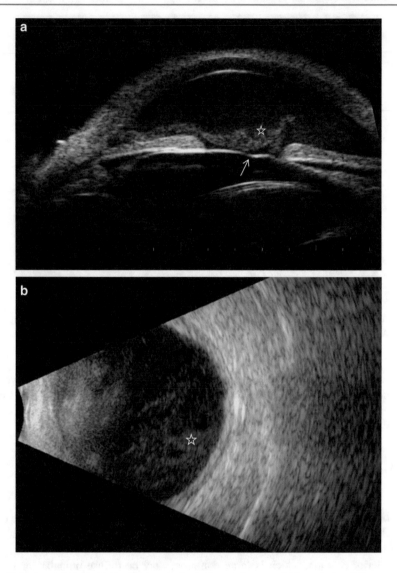

Fig. 7.25 A case of phacolytic glaucoma: **a** Irregular anterior capsule (arrow) denoting rupture of
the anterior capsule with leakage of the lens matter into the anterior chamber (star), **b** B-scan
showing multiple echoes in the vitreous cavity denoting vitritis (star)

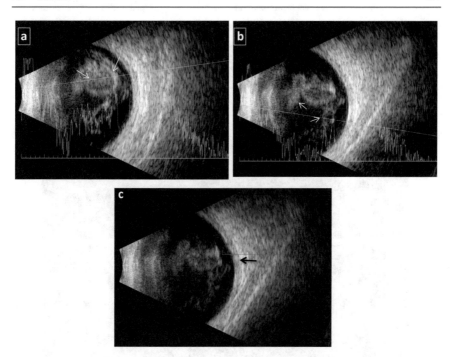

Fig. 7.26 A case of postoperative cataract showing, **a** dislocated lens fragments (white arrows) in the vitreous cavity with moderate irregular reflectivity in A-scan, **b** surrounded with multiple echoes and membranes (white arrows) of variable irregular reflectivity in A-scan, **c** evidence of choroidal thickening (Black arrow)

7.9.1 Diffuse Scleritis

UBM of diffuse anterior scleritis appears as mottled internal reflectivity with areas of lower reflectivity scattered throughout the involved region. The diffuse mottling represents scleral infiltration with inflammatory cells and edema of collagen bundles.

Ultrasound of diffuse posterior scleritis appears as thickening of the sclera, which can vary in degree and can be either diffuse or localized. Usually, the thickened sclera is highly reflective, with regular internal structure. Thickening of the retinochoroidal layer can also be observed, associated with swelling of underlying Tenon's capsule and episclera causing an echolucent area (Figs. 7.31, 7.32, 7.33, and 7.34). When peripapillary in location this causes a 'T' sign appearance [40] (Figs. 7.35 and 7.36).

Exudative retinal and choroidal detachment, optic nerve edema and nerve sheath edema may also be seen.

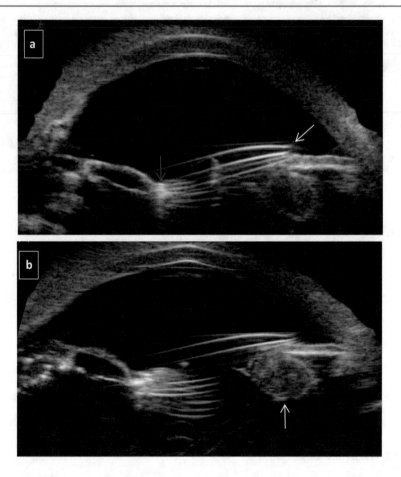

Fig. 7.27 UBM of a case of pupillary capture IOL causing recurrent postoperative inflammation, **a** revealing one edge of the IOL impacted in the pupillary edge of the iris (red arrow) at one side and the opposite edge of the IOL above the anterior surface of the iris at the pupillary edge (white arrow) **b** evidence of Soemmerring's ring (arrow)

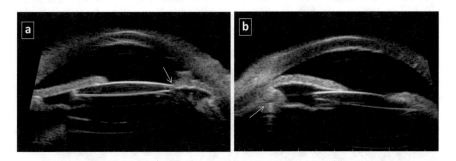

Fig. 7.28 UBM of a case of a decentered IOL, **a** IOL pushed anteriorly with one edge of the IOL pushing the pupillary margin (white arrow) of the iris causing iris bombe (red arrow) at this side, **b** the IOL haptic pressing on the ciliary body

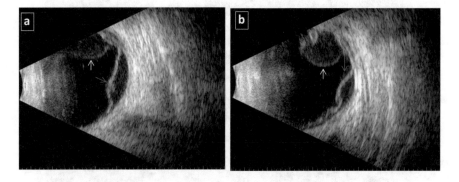

Fig. 7.29 **a** Longitudinal B-scan of the same patient showing multiple echoes of low amplitude collapsed anteriorly denoting vitritis (white arrows) with exudative retinal detachment (red arrow) **b** longitudinal B-scan revealing the detached retina anteriorly

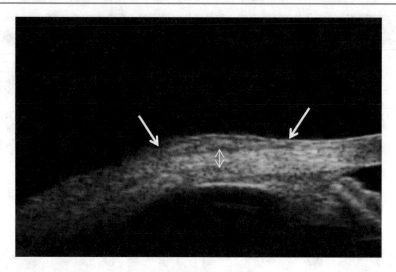

Fig. 7.30 Nodular episcleritis with moderate reflectivity (arrows representing margins of the nodule), without invovment of the scleral layer(double arrows)

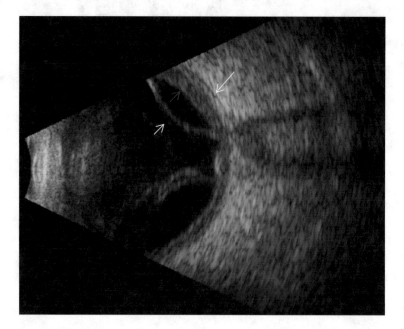

Fig. 7.31 A case of posterior scleritis with serous retinal detachment (white arrow), choroidal thickening (red arrow)and scleral thickening with mild oedema of the sub-Tenon's space (black arrow)

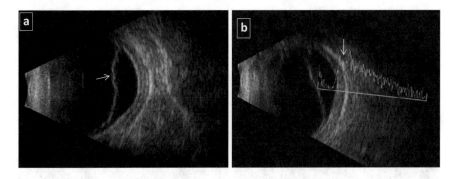

Fig. 7.32 A case of posterior scleritis, **a** scleral thickening and choroidal thickening with secondary retinal detachment(white arrow), **b** showing the high reflectivity of the choroid and sclera followed by decreased reflectivity of the superimposed arbitrary A-scan due to infiltration of the sub-Tenon's capsule (white arrow)

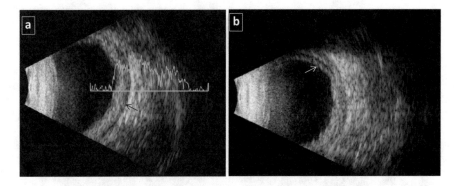

Fig. 7.33 **a** Transverse B-scan showing diffuse thickening of the scleral layer with high regular internal reflectivity on A-scan with oedema of the sub-Tenon's space (black arrow), **b** Longitudinal scan exposing the periphery showing ciliochoroidal detachment

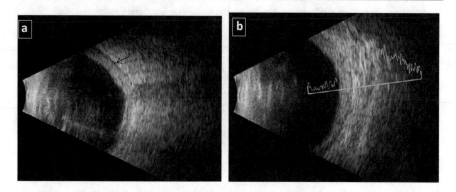

Fig. 7.34 a Axial B-scan demonstrating retinochoroidal thickening and scleral thickening with oedema in the sub-Tenon's space (black arrows in **a** and **b**), **b** Superimposed A-scan of the sclera of high amplitude with regular internal reflectivity

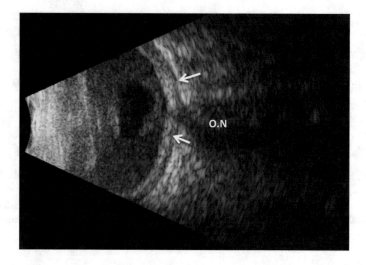

Fig. 7.35 Axial scan of T-sign with diffuse scleral thickening and distension of the sub-Tenon's space(white arrows) around the optic nerve(O.D)

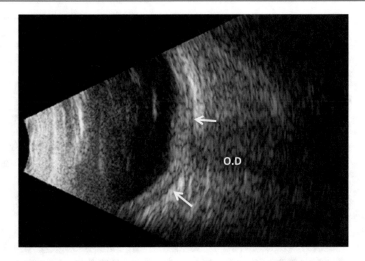

Fig. 7.36 Another patient with flattened ocular contour in an axial B-scan of T-sign with diffuse scleral thickening and distension of the sub-Tenon's space (white arrows)around the optic disc (O. D)

7.9.2 Nodular and Necrotic Scleritis

*The UBM of nodular anterior scleritis appear as thickened episclera with localized nodule of lower reflectivity than the surrounding sclera [41] (Fig. 7.37) and in Necrotizing scleritis there will be a scleral thinning (Fig. 7.38).

*Nodular posterior scleritis can present as an elevated choroidal mass resembling an intraocular tumor. The thickened sclera in these nodular lesions demonstrates high reflectivity with regular internal structure on ultrasonography [43, 44].

Choroidal and ciliary body detachments, as well as ciliochoroidal effusion syndrome may also occur in the setting of posterior scleritis and can be confirmed by ultrasonography (Figs. 7.36 and 7.38).

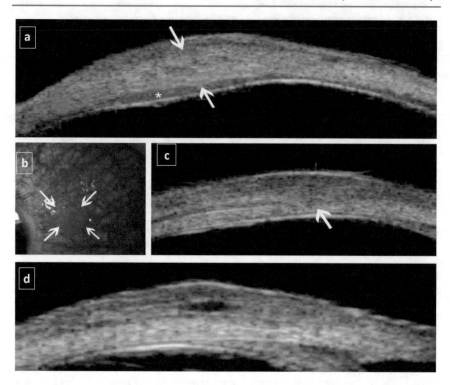

Fig. 7.37 Nodular Scleritis. **a** Left eye nodular scleritis. Ultrasound biomicroscopy (UBM) show-ing a circumscribed area of non-homogenous scleral thickening (arrows) with an irregular upper surface and inner small hyporeflective areas. Note also mild underlying choroidal swelling (*). **b–d** Another patient with Bilateral nodular scleritis. Left eye: **b** clinical photograph showing a temporal scleral nodule (arrows) with oedema and congestion of superficial and deep episcleral vessels. **c** UBM showing a focal area of scleral thickening and irregularity of the upper scleral surface. Right eye: **d** UBM showing a focal area of scleral thickening and irregularity of the upper scleral surface with a hyporeflective fluid pocket. (Zur, Dinah, et al. "High-resolution ultrasound biomicroscopy as an adjunctive diagnostic tool for anterior scleral inflammatory disease." Acta ophthalmologica) [42]

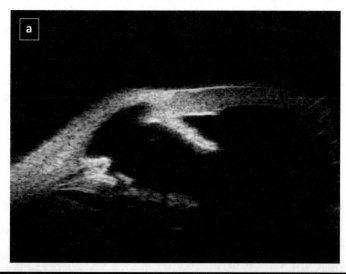

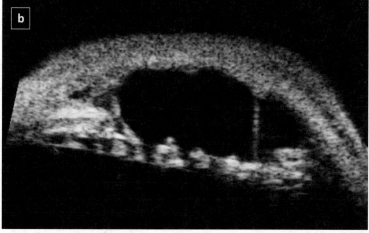

Fig. 7.38 Longitudnal UBM scan in a case of necrotizing scleritis (**a**) the sclera is barely seen with evidence of anterior staphyloma, (**b**) transverse UBM scan of the necrotized sclera

References

1. Moschos MM, Yan G-C. Anterior segment granuloma and optic nerve involvement as the presenting signs of systemic sarcoidosis. Clin Ophthalmol (auckland, Nz). 2008;2(4):951–3.
2. Robert R, Pogorelov P, Mardin CY, Szkaradek M, Juenemann AGM. Solitary sarcoid granuloma of the Iris mimicking tuberculosis: a case report. J Ophthalmol. 2014; Article ID 656042, 3 pages, 2014. https://doi.org/10.1155/2014/656042.
3. Yang P. Auxiliary ocular examinations. In: Atlas of uveitis. Singapore: Springer; 2021. https://doi.org/10.1007/978-981-15-3726-4_5.

4. Peizeng Y, et al. Longitudinal study of anterior segment inflammation by ultrasound biomicroscopy in patients with acute anterior uveitis. Acta Ophthalmol. 2009;87(2):211–5.
5. Ahn, Jae Kyoun, and In Young Jeong. Ultrasound biomicroscopy in anterior uveitis. Ophthalmology 115.10 (2008): 1851–1851.
6. Pichi F, Srivastava SK. Optical coherence tomography evaluation of the anterior segment in uveitis patients. In: Multimodal imaging in uveitis. Cham: Springer; 2018. p. 99–106.
7. Tran VT, LeHoang P, Herbort CP. Value of high-frequency ultrasound biomicroscopy in uveitis. Eye. 2001;15(1):23–30.
8. Lin W, Beardsley RM, Skalet AH, Wilson DJ, Rosenbaum JT, Lin P. Bilateral Idiopathic solitary granuloma of the uveal tract: diagnosis and treatment. Int J Ophthalmic Pathol. 2015;4 (4):166. https://doi.org/10.4172/2324-8599.1000166. Epub 2015 Oct 15. PMID: 26779545; PMCID: PMC4711913.
9. Bonfioli AA, et al. Intermediate uveitis. Semin Ophthalmol. 2005;20(3). Taylor & Francis, 2005.
10. Greiner KH, et al. Grading of pars planitis by ultrasound biomicroscopy—echographic and clinical study. Eur J Ultrasound. 2002;15(3):139–44.
11. Oksala A. Ultrasonic findings in the vitreous body in patients with acute anterior uveitis. Acta Ophthalmol. 1977;55(2):287–93.
12. Häring G, Nölle B, Wiechens B. Ultrasound biomicroscopic imaging in intermediate uveitis. Br J Ophthalmol. 1998;82(6):625–9.
13. Doro D, et al. Combined 50-and 20-MHz frequency ultrasound imaging in intermediate uveitis. Am J Ophthalmol. 2006;141(5):953–5.
14. Biswas J, Bhende MP, Mondkar SV. Ultrasound biomicroscopy in anterior segment inflammatory disorders. Ann Ophthalmol. 2000;32(4):301–6.
15. Nussenblatt RB, et al. Standardizatlon of Vitreal inflammatory activity in intermediate and posterior uveitis. Ophthalmology. 1985;92(4):467–71.
16. Descheˆnes J, Mansour M, Rudzinski M. Ultrasound and ultrasound biomicroscopy as a diagnostic tool. Dev Ophthalmol. 1999;31:14–21.
17. Yannuzzi NA, Si N, Relhan N, Kuriyan AE, Albini TA, Berrocal AM, Davis JL, Smiddy WE, Townsend J, Miller D, Flynn Jr. HW, Endophthalmitis After Clear Corneal Cataract Surgery: Outcomes Over Two Decades, American Journal of Ophthalmology (2016), doi: https://doi.org/10.1016/j.ajo.2016.11.006
18. Arora R, et al. Bilateral endogenous panophthalmitis caused by Salmonella typhi: first case report. Orbit. 2008;27(2):115–7.
19. Haripriya A, et al. Nocardia endophthalmitis after cataract surgery: clinicomicrobiological study. Am J Ophthalmol. 2005;139(5):837–46.
20. Byrne SF. Ultrasound of the eye and orbit. Mosby Incorporated; 2002.
21. Kohanim S, et al. Utility of ocular ultrasonography in diagnosing infectious endophthalmitis in patients with media opacities. Semin Ophthalmol. 2012;27(5–6). Taylor & Francis, 2012.
22. Patil R, et al. Relationship of echographic findings with visual outcomes in post-cataract surgery endophthalmitis. Ann Ophthalmol. 2004;36(1):12–16.
23. Ahn JK. Morphologic changes in the anterior segment in patients with initial-onset or recurrent Vogt-Koyanagi-Harada disease. Ocul Immunol Inflamm. 2010;18(4):314–8.
24. Attia S, Khochtali S, Kahloun R, Ammous D, Jelliti B, Ben Yahia S, Zaouali S, Khairallah M. Clinical and multimodal imaging characteristics of acute Vogt-Koyanagi-Harada disease unassociated with clinically evident exudative retinal detachment. Int Ophthalmol. 2016;36 (1):37–44. https://doi.org/10.1007/s10792-015-0073-7 Epub 2015 May 5 PMID: 25939987.
25. Yeh J-P, et al. Point-of-care ultrasound diagnosis of bilateral retinal detachment associated with Vogt-Koyanagi-Harada disease in the pediatric emergency department. Pediatr Emerg Care. 2016;32(9):639–41.
26. Bhende M, et al. Atlas of ophthalmic ultrasound and ultrasound biomicroscopy. JP Medical Ltd; 2013.

27. Cella W, et al. Ultrasound biomicroscopy findings in peripheral vitreoretinal toxocariasis. Eur J Ophthalmol. 2004;14(2):132–6.
28. Chen Q, et al. Role of ultrasound biomicroscopy in diagnosis of ocular toxocariasis. Br J Ophthalmol. 2018;102(5):642–6.
29. Liu J, et al. Ultrasound biomicroscopic imaging in paediatric ocular toxocariasis. Br J Ophthalmol. 2017;101(11):1514–17.
30. Dhiman R, Devi S, Duraipandi K, Chandra P, Vanathi M, Tandon R, Sen S. Cysticercosis of the eye. Int J Ophthalmol. 2017;10(8):1319–24.
31. Pujari A, Chawla R, Singh R, et al. Ultrasound-B scan: an indispensable tool for diagnosing ocular cysticercosis. Case Rep. 2017;2017:bcr-2017-219346.
32. Sharma T, et al. Intraocular cysticercosis: clinical characteristics and visual outcome after vitreoretinal surgery. Ophthalmology. 2003;110(5):996–1004.
33. Das D, et al. Neuro and intraocular cysticercosis: a clinicopathological case report. Eye Brain. 2010;2:39.
34. Raval V, Khetan V. Spectral domain optical coherence tomography features of subretinal cysticercus cyst. J Ophthalmic Vis Res. 2012;7(4):347.
35. Ganesh SK, Priyanka. Analysis of clinical profile, investigation, and management of ocular cysticercosis seen at a tertiary referral centre. Ocul Immunol Inflamm. 2018;26(4):550–7.
36. Pushker N, Bajaj MS, Betharia SM. Orbital and adnexal cysticercosis. Clin Experiment Ophthalmol. 2002;30:322–33. https://doi.org/10.1046/j.1442-9071.2002.00550.x.
37. Piette S, et al. Ultrasound biomicroscopy in uveitis-glaucoma-hyphema syndrome. Am J Ophthalmol. 2002;133(6):839–41.
38. Suwan Y, et al. Pseudophakic angle-closure from a Soemmering ring. BMC Ophthalmol. 2016;16(1):91.
39. Bhatt DC. Ultrasound biomicroscopy: an overview. J Clin Ophthalmol Res. 2014;2(2):115.
40. Ciardella AP, et al. Imaging techniques for posterior uveitis. Curr Opin Ophthalmol. 2004;15 (6):519–30.
41. Pavlin CJ, Stuart Foster F. Ultrasound biomicroscopy of the eye. Springer Science & Business Media; 2012.
42. Zur D, et al. High resolution ultrasound biomicroscopy as an adjunctive diagnostic tool for anterior scleral inflammatory disease. Acta Ophthalmol. 2016;94(6):e384–9.
43. Moreira-Neto C, et al. Nodular posterior scleritis associated with presumed ocular tuberculosis: a multimodal imaging case report. Am J Ophthalmol Case Rep. 2019;16:100558.
44. Alsarhani WK, Abu El-Asrar AM. Multimodal imaging of nodular posterior scleritis: Case report and review of the literature. Middle East Afr J Ophthalmol. 2020;27(2):134.

Glaucoma

8

8.1 Angle Closure Glaucoma

In angle closure glaucoma, forces are generated to cause angle closure in four anatomic sites: the iris (pupillary block), the ciliary body (plateau iris), the lens (phacomorphic glaucoma), and behind the iris by a combination of various forces (malignant glaucoma) [1, 48].

UBM provides valuable information that can help differentiating these affected sites and can greatly assist in choosing the effective line of treatment [51, 53] (Fig. 8.1).

8.1.1 Pupillary Block

In pupillary block glaucoma, the iris assumes a convex profile (forward bowing of iris) due to the pressure differential between the posterior and anterior chambers [2, 3].

The anterior convexity of the iris lifts the iris off the lens surface to the point where only the tip of the iris is lying against the lens surface, this amount of lens-iris contact is less than that seen in normal eyes. The iris convexity increases the distance of the iris from the zonule and peripheral lens providing a margin of safety for Yag laser iridotomy [4, 35].

© The Author(s), under exclusive license to Springer Nature Switzerland AG 2021 213
R. Abbas, *Ophthalmic Ultrasonography and Ultrasound Biomicroscopy*,
https://doi.org/10.1007/978-3-030-76979-6_8

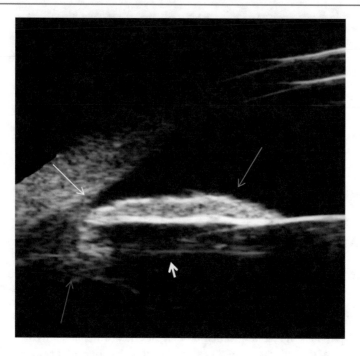

Fig. 8.1 UBM image of a normal eye showing the angle. The iris (blue arrow), scleral spur (white thin arrow), zonules (short white arrow) and ciliary process (red arrow)

A shallow anterior chamber, and narrow angle recess are characteristic findings in the UBM of pupillary block glaucoma. Some eyes may have associated ciliary effusion [20, 41]. In majority of pupillary block glaucoma cases, the ciliary sulcus is open, with a space between the ciliary processes and the back of the iris [4, 52] (Figs. 8.2, 8.3 and 8.4).

Fig. 8.2 Longitudinal UBM
scan of Right and Left eye
showing bilateral pupillary
block with anterior iris
bowing(blue arrows) and slit
opening of the angle (white
arrows) with more obliterated
angle recess in the Left eye

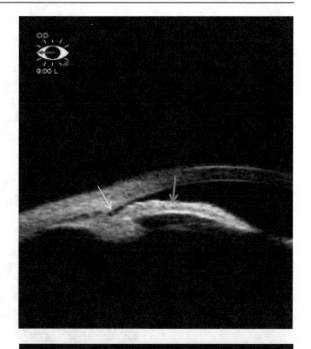

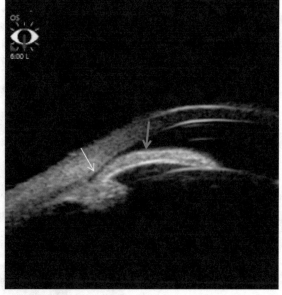

Fig. 8.3 A case of bilateral pupillary block, longitudinal UBM scan of the Right and Left eye showing shallow anterior chamber (double arrow) with anterior iris bowing obliterating the angle (black arrows)

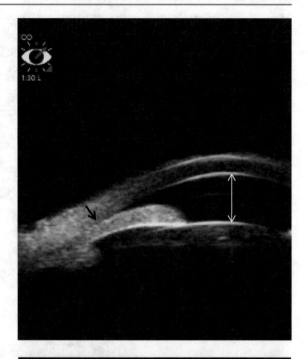

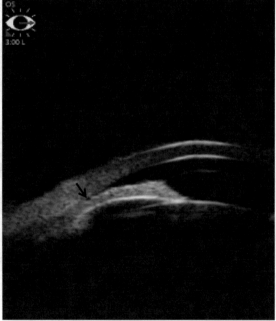

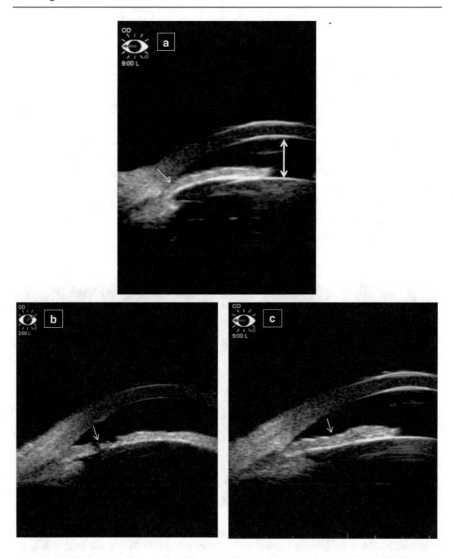

Fig. 8.4 a A case of pupillary block prior to iridotomy showing anterior iris bowing oblitrating the angle (white arrow), shallow anterior chamber (double arrow) and opened ciliary sulcus(red arrow), **b** showing patent peripheral iridotomy (PI) (arrow), **c** The iris profile becomes a straight line after the Peripheral iridotomy (arrow)

8.1.2   Plateau Iris

In plateau iris the ciliary processes are anteriorly located, closing the ciliary sulcus, and providing structural support behind the peripheral iris [23]. A good way of looking at this phenomenon is that the ciliary processes and the trabecular mesh-work form a port through which the iris thickness must pass [2]. The smaller this port and/or the thicker the iris in this region, the greater the degree of angle closure.

The iris surface looks flat or slightly convex just like in a normal eye [1]. It can also confirm the "double hump sign" which is normally seen with gonioscopy by the use of an indentation. UBM special technique that imposes mild pressure on peripheral cornea with the skirt of the eyecup [5, 31].

UBM can provide other evidence of plateau iris such small anterior chamber depth, absence of trabecular-ciliary process distance, as well as iris-zonule distance that is smaller than normal (Figs. 8.5 and 8.6).

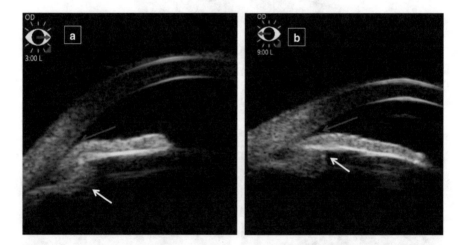

Fig. 8.5 Longitudinal UBM scans of temporal and nasal side (at 3 and 9 o'clock), showing a case of Plateau iris. Note the anterior location of the ciliary processes (white arrow in **a**) closing the ciliary sulcus (white arrow in **b**), and preventing the peripheral iris from falling away from the trabecular meshwork and narrowing the angle (Red arrows)

Fig. 8.6 Longitudinal UBM scan of Plateau iris showing the double hump sign on indentation

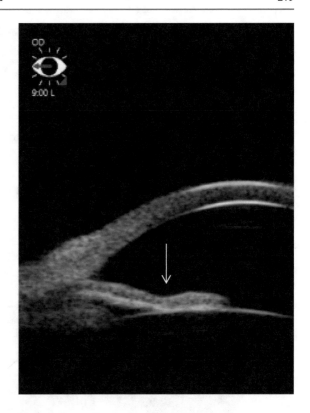

8.1.3 Malignant Glaucoma

Malignant glaucoma is defined as a condition in which shallowing of the anterior chamber with elevated pressure occurs in spite of a patent iridotomy. Also known as aqueous misdirection or ciliary block. Malignant glaucoma usually occurs after glaucoma surgeries; however, it can also occur after other ocular interventions such as phacoemulsification, laser iridotomy, laser capsulotomy or cyclophotocoagulation [6, 18, 29].

Although the exact etiology of this disease is not yet fully understood, it is believed to evolve from posterior misdirection of the aqueous humor into or behind the vitreous. The resultant pressure differential between the posterior and anterior chambers causes an anterior displacement of the lens-iris diaphragm, anterior chamber shallowing or flattening, and secondary angle closure glaucoma [7, 45, 46].

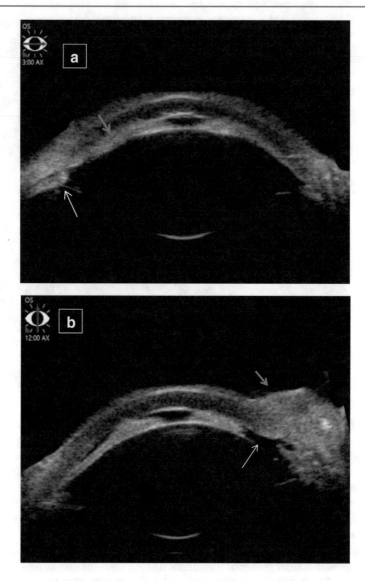

Fig. 8.7 **a** Axial UBM scan of flat anterior chamber with forward movement of the iris-lens diaphragm causing iridocorneal touch (blue arrow), and ciliary body rotation (white arrow), **b** showing thickened conjunctival bleb (blue arrow), with patent Peripheral iridectomy (white arrow)

UBM findings include shallow or flat anterior chamber, anterior rotation of ciliary processes. Supraciliary effusion may or may not be present. The detection of supraciliary effusion on UBM is of significance as it indicates the need for aggressive medical management rather than immediate surgical intervention [8] (Figs. 8.7 and 8.8).

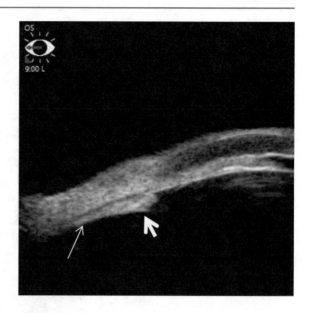

Fig. 8.8 Longitudinal UBM scan showing the anteriorly rotated ciliary body (thick arrow) with no evidence of ciliochoroidal detachment (thin arrow)

8.2 Open Angle Glaucoma

Although UBM can provide a clear, objective view of the anterior segment, its utility is limited in open angle glaucoma because changes taking place in open angle glaucoma occur at a level beyond the current resolution of ultrasound biomicroscopy.

8.2.1 Pigment Dispersion Syndrome

In pigment dispersion syndrome, friction between the posterior iris surface and the anterior zonular bundles causes the disintegration of iris pigment epithelial cells and the release of pigment granules, which are then dispersed by aqueous currents. The liberated pigment is deposited throughout the anterior segment. The classic diagnostic triad consists of a Krukenberg spindle, slitlike radial midperipheral iris transillumination defects, and increased pigmentation of the trabecular meshwork [9, 16].

In UBM the angles are widely open. The iris is with slight concavity (bowing posteriorly), as is true in pupillary block, there is a relative pressure gradient between the anterior and posterior chamber; however, because the anterior chamber is the one that holds higher pressure, this condition is called "reverse pupillary block" [1, 38] (Fig. 8.9).

Fig. 8.9 Pigmentary glaucoma; UBM of an eye with pigment dispersion syndrome. **a** Note the deep anterior chamber(double head arrow), concave iris (white arrows), **b** Iridozonular touch (blue arrow), **c** multiple echoes in the anterior chamber of low amplitude on A-scan

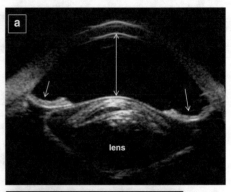

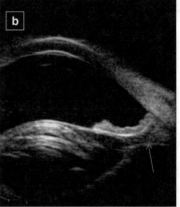

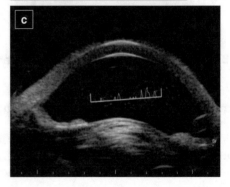

8.3 UBM in Assessing Efficacy of Therapy

8.3.1 Laser Peripheral Iridotomy

laser peripheral iridotomy, (PI) imaged as a much more irregular opening, with stromal disruption compared to surgical iridectomy. The most important use of UBM post PI is the identification of anterior rotation of ciliary processes and absence of ciliary sulcus to identify plateau iris. The presence of cysts of the ciliary processes may be seen [8] (Figs. 8.10 and 8.11).

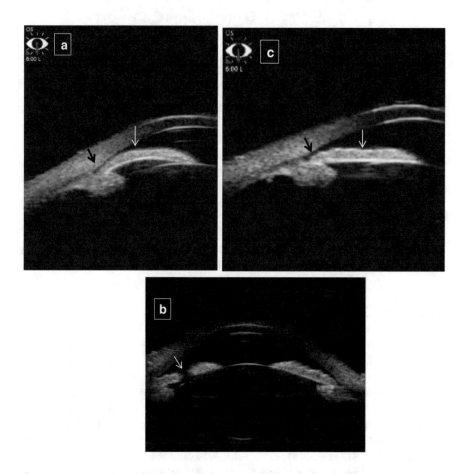

Fig. 8.10 A case of pupil block glaucoma **a** longitudinal scan of the inferior quadrant showing convex iris bowing (white arrow), slit-like opening of the angle (black arrow) and opened ciliary sulcus, **b** axial scan showing patent peripheral iridotomy(white arrow) at 12 o'clock, **c** The iris profile becomes a straight line at the inferior quadrant (white arrow) with change in the angle opening distance(black arrow)

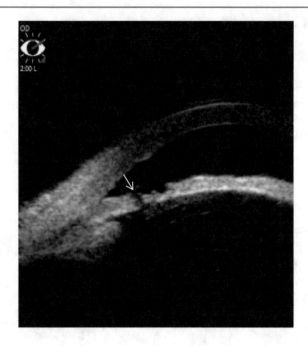

Fig. 8.11   A longitudinal UBM scan of Patent Peripheral iridotomy shows irregular iris stromal disruption (white arrow)

8.3.2   Surgical Iridectomy

*Surgical iridectomy sites generally show a smooth edged gap in the iris on ultrasound biomicroscopy (Figs. 8.12a, 8.14c, and 8.15a).

8.3.3   Post-Glaucoma Surgery

The basic mechanism of trabeculectomy is to create a fistula at the limbus allowing aqueous humor to drain from the anterior chamber to the episcleral and subconjunctival spaces, thereby reducing the intraocular pressure (IOP) [10, 37].

UBM identifies the status of a filtering bleb; the height, internal reflectivity within the bleb, cysts inside the bleb and patency of the stoma and its connection to the bleb [32, 33]. The UBM images of eyes with good IOP control are characterized by better visibility of the route under the scleral flap and a low reflectivity inside the bleb [8, 17, 25–28] (Figs. 8.11, 8.12, 8.13, 8.14, and 8.15).

The most popular non penetrating filtering procedures involve removal of a deep scleral flap, the external wall of Schlemm's canal and corneal stroma behind the anterior trabeculum and Descemet's membrane, thus creating an intrascleral space. The aqueous humor leaves the anterior chamber through the intact trabeculo-Descemet's membrane into the scleral space [11, 21, 34, 36].

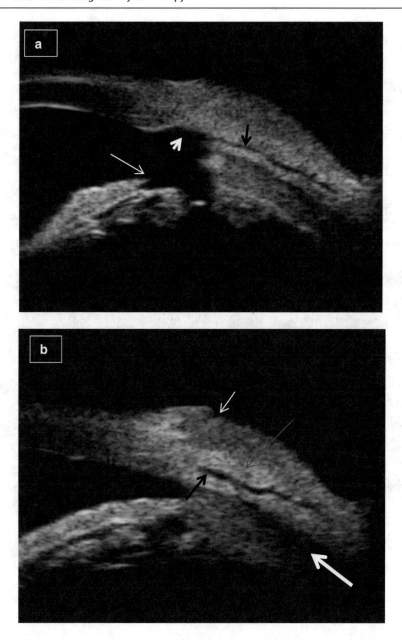

Fig. 8.12 Post trabeculectomy showing **a** A Patent ostium (short white arrow) and peripheral iridectomy (thin arrow)with patent intrascleral pathway (black arrow in **a** and **b**), **b** Elevated bleb with low echogenicity (thin white arrow) above the patent intrascleral pathway(black arrow), with evidence of intrableb microcysts. Note the supraciliary effusion(thick white arrow), scleral flap (red arrow)

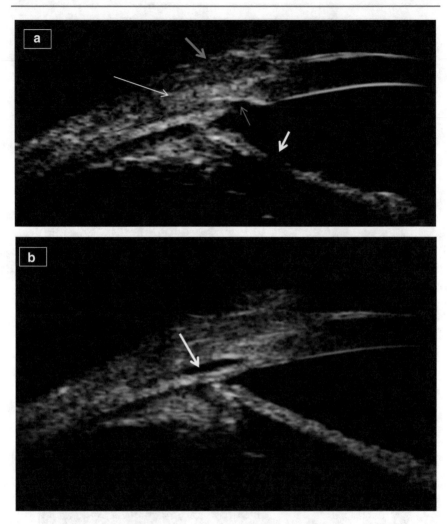

Fig. 8.13 Post trabeculectomy **a** A patent ostium(thin blue arrow) with intrascleral tract (red arrow), peripheral iridectomy (short white arrow)and evident scleral flap (long white arrow), with formed low echogenic bleb (thick blue arrow), **b** showing patent intrasleral tract (white Arrow)

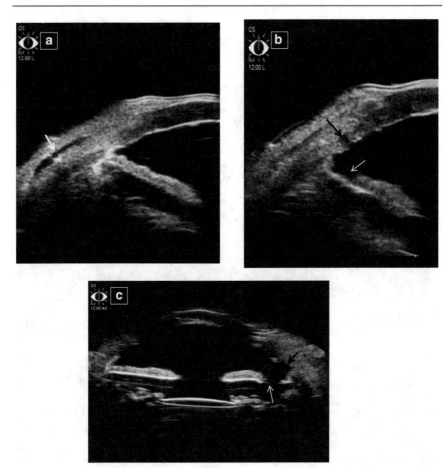

Fig. 8.14 a Magnified longitudinal UBM scan of a diffuse filtrating bleb; the bleb showing opened fluid space (white arrow), **b** showing the ostium with peripheral iridectomy. **c** Axial UBM scan of the same patient showing the peripheral iridectomy (white arrow), and the ostium (black arrow)

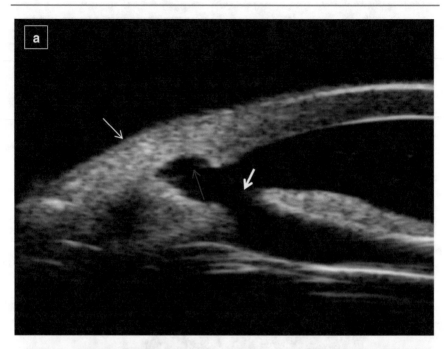

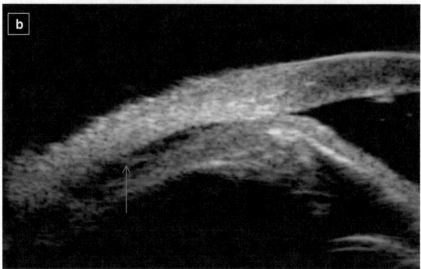

Fig. 8.15 Post trabeculectomy. **a** Longitudinal UBM scan showing the ostium (red arrow) with no evident of scleral tract with flat bleb (white arrow), as well as peripheral iridectomy (short thick arrow), **b** evident of ciliochoroidal detachment (blue arrow)

UBM examination can demonstrate the presence of intrascleral space and the remaining thin TDM (trabeculo-descemet's membrane) and a filtering bleb (Fig. 8.16).

Associated features like suprachoroidal effusion and ciliary process rotation can be detected by UBM (Fig. 8.17).

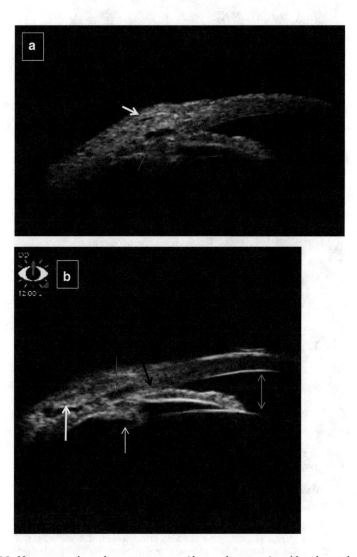

Fig. 8.16 Non penetrating glaucoma surgery (deep sclerectomy): with adequately formed intrascleral space (red arrow in **a** and **b**), and evidence of formed bleb of low echogenicity with evident of fluid space (short white arrow), **b** Apparent scleral flap (white arrow) with visible trabeculo-descemet's membrane (black arrow). Note the iris in contact with the TDM, Moreover, the UBM scan is showing evidence of anterior rotation of the ciliary body (thin white arrow)and shallow anterior chamber (double head arrow)

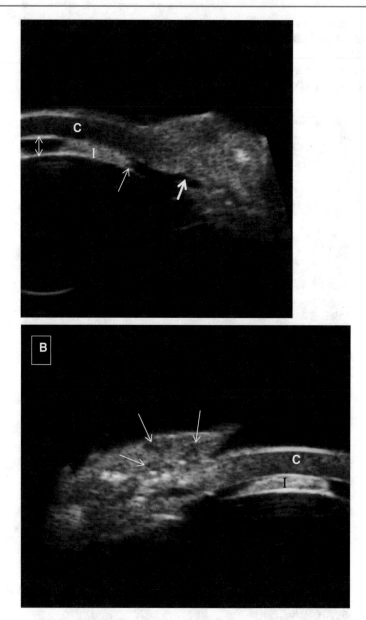

Fig. 8.17 A case of malignant glaucoma **a** showing patent ostium (thick arrows) with peripheral iridectomy (thin arrow), **b** Elevated low to moderate echogenic bleb with microcysts (arrows). Note the flat anterior chamber with forward movement of the iris-lens diaphragm and the iridocorneal touch (double arrow in **a**), C:cornea, I: iris,

8.3.4 Glaucoma Implants (Tubes, Tube Shunts, Valves)

The patency of aqueous drainage tubes as well as the location can be determined by
UBM [40]. Where A&B-scan ultrasonography may be used to identify the presence
or absence of a glaucoma filtering bleb over the glaucoma implant plate especially
if the plate is sutured into place at or posterior to the ocular equator [19, 24, 30, 39]
(Figs. 8.18, 8.19, 8.20 and 8.21).

Fig. 8.18 **a** and
b Longitudinal UBM scan
showing implanted tube in the
anterior chamber, I (iris), T
(Tube), **c** Transverse B-scan
showing a patent superior
"Ahmed glaucoma drainage
device" with large fluid
reservoir (black arrow)

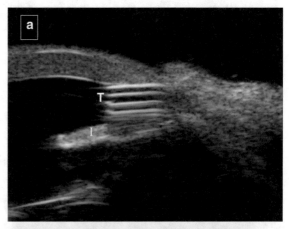

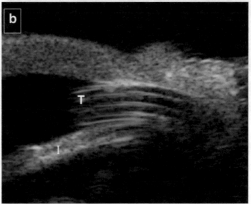

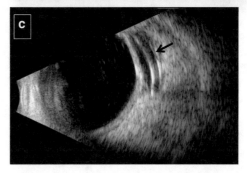

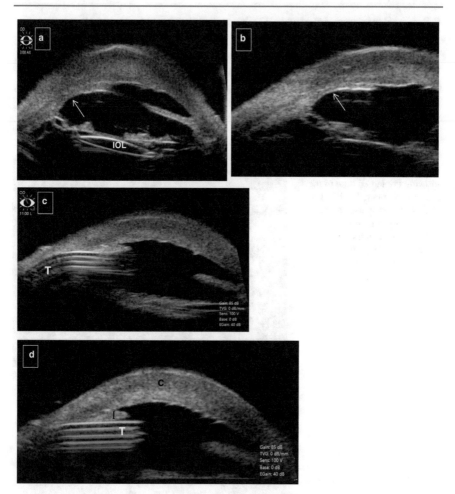

Fig. 8.19 **a** and **b** Axial and longitudinal UBM scan of an eye with anterior synechiae (white arrow) at 9 o'clock extending to 12 o'clock. Note the tilted IOL. **c** and **d** Implanted tube in the posterior chamber with the iris seen above it (I: iris), (c: cornea), (T: tube)

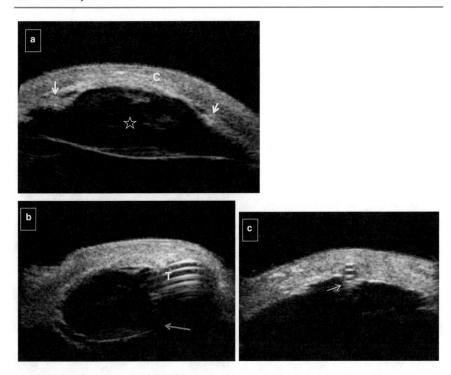

Fig. 8.20 a A case with total anterior synechiae (short arrows) showing the lens (star) pushed anteriorly causing lenticulo-corneal touch (c: cornea), **b** The implanted tube obliterated by the lens (arrow), **c** transverse scan exposing the obliterated tube

8.4   Secondary Glaucoma

The estimated proportion of glaucoma damage that is clearly secondary to other ocular or systemic disease, or to trauma, may represent as much as 20% of all glaucoma subtypes. Secondary glaucoma is properly considered to represent those

Fig. 8.21 Transverse B-scan
of different patients showing
patent superior glaucoma
drainage devices with large
fluid reservoir (arrows)

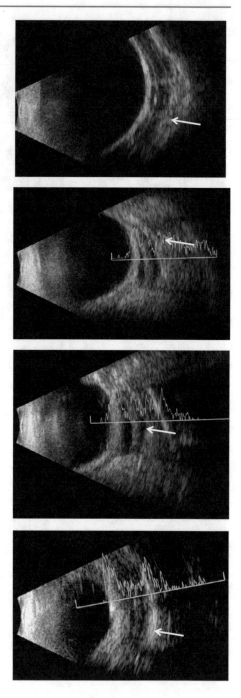

eyes in which a second form of ocular pathology has caused IOP above the normal range, leading to optic nerve damage [12, 49, 50] (Figs. 8.22, 8.23, 8.24, 8.25, 8.26, 8.27, 8.28, 8.29, 8.30 and 8.31). These processes may include one of the following:

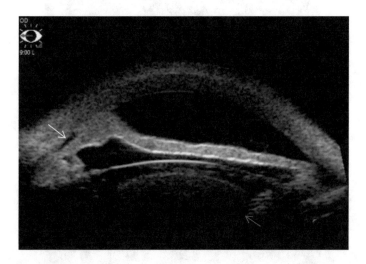

Fig. 8.22 UBM scan of a case of uveitis showing peripheral anterior synechiae with aqueous-filled slit-like opening (white arrow). Note the swollen cataractous lens (red arrow)

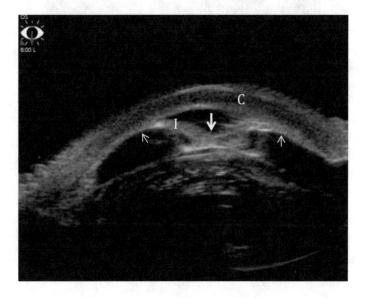

Fig. 8.23 Axial UBM scan of occlusio pupillea (thick arrow) with iris bombe causing iridocorneal adhesion (short arrows) leading to angle obliteration. (C: cornea—I: iris)

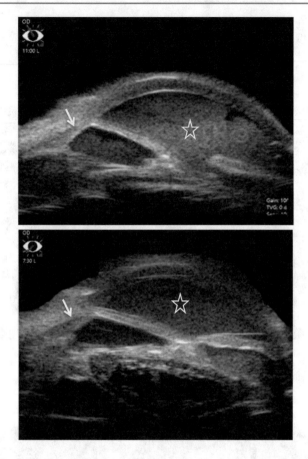

Fig. 8.24 A case of hyphema (star) with anterior synechiae (white arrow) obliterating the angle almost in all quadrants

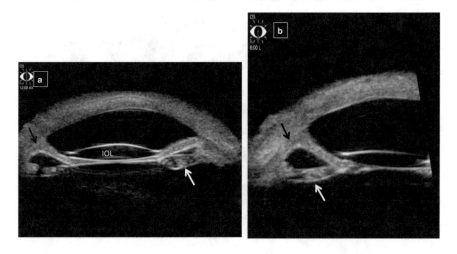

Fig. 8.25 a and **b** Axial and Longitudinal UBM scans showing pupillary IOL capture causing anterior synechiae obliterating the angle (black arrows), Note the Soemmering's ring (white arrows)

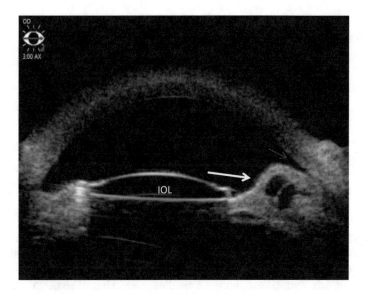

Fig. 8.26 Axial UBM scan of pupillary IOL capture causing iris cyst formation (white arrow) almost oblitrating the angle (red arrow)

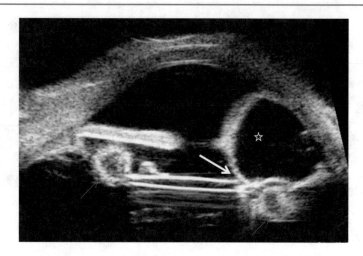

Fig. 8.27 A case of a sublaxated IOL with the haptic embedded in the iris (white arrow) causing iris irritation and cyst formation (star) resulting in oblitration of the angle at this site. Note the soemoering's ring formation at both sides (red arrows)

(1) Neovascularization
(2) Uveitic
(3) Trauma
(4) Lens related.

8.5 Congenital Glaucoma

Primary congenital glaucoma (PCG), the most common primary childhood glaucoma, is believed to be caused by dysplasia of the anterior chamber angle, and it is generally bilateral [13].

The eyes of congenital glaucoma patients are known to have greater corneal diameters, greater axial length, and higher myopic refractive error. Along with features of significantly increased corneal diameters and increased axial length, thinned out iris and ciliary body anomalies were characteristic of congenital glaucoma [14, 22, 42, 47].

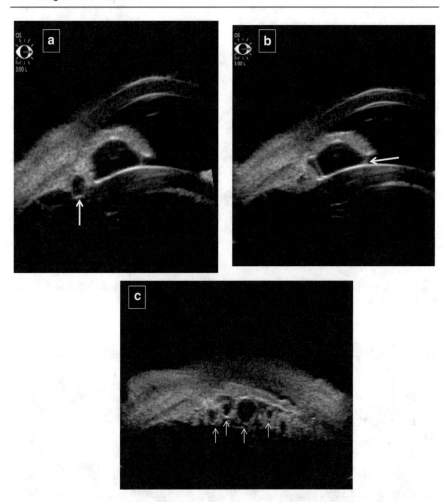

Fig. 8.28 a and **b** Longitudinal UBM scan showing multiloculated multiple cyst (white arrows) pushing the iris forward and closing the angle (red arrows). **c** A transvrese UBM scan demostrating the multiple cysts of different sizes (white arrows)

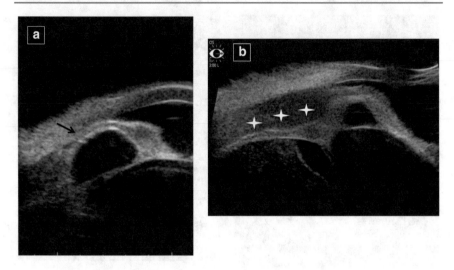

Fig. 8.29 Longitudinal UBM scans of a patient with uveal effusion syndrome. Note the oblitrated angle seen in (**a**) and supraciliary effusion (stars) seen in (**b**)

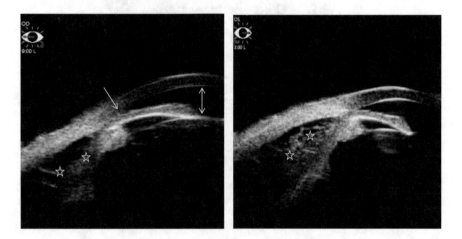

Fig. 8.30 Longitudinal UBM Scan of bilateral uveal effusion syndrome. Note the closed angle (white arrow) and supraciliary effusion (stars). Note the shallow anterior chamber (double arrow)

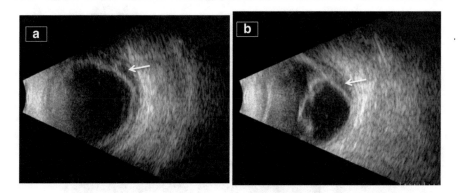

Fig. 8.31 **a** and **b** B-scan of the same patient in different quadrant showing ciliochoroidal detachment extending posteriorly with suprachoroidal effusion (white arrows)

UBM of primary congenital glaucoma include:

Thin cornea with larger diameter, deep anterior chamber, narrow posterior chamber, reduced iris thickness, wide anterior chamber angle, absence of iris crypts which is probably caused by lack of iris sphincter and dilator muscle, although uveal and neuroepithelial layers are preserved, possible anterior iris insertion or abnormal angle membrane (thin hyperreflective membrane that covers angle structures can be visible (Barkan's membrane), and ciliary process abnormalities [43] (Figs. 8.32, 8.33, 8.34, 8.35, 8.36, 8.37 and 8.38).

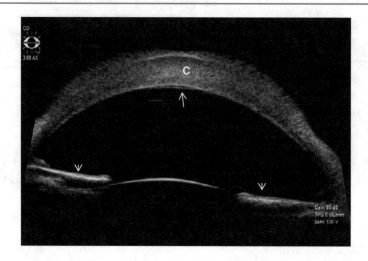

Fig. 8.32 **a** Axial UBM scan of the right eye showing thickened cornea with increased corneal diameter, thin flat iris with loss of iris crypts(short arrows), with Descemet's membrane breaks (white arrow). (C: cornea)

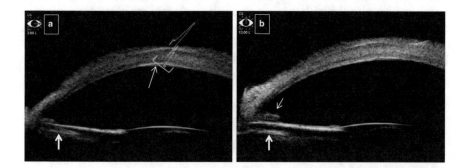

Fig. 8.33 UBM scans of the left eye of the same Patient, **a** showing the same findings of the Right eye in Fig. 8.32, with the superimposed A-scan of the breaks of Descemet''s membrane (white arrow)and with thin stretched-out ciliary body(thick arrow in **a** and **b**), **b** showing an abnormal membrane in the angle

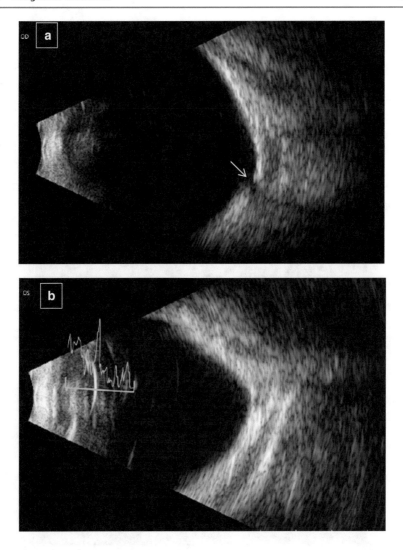

Fig. 8.34 B-scan of the same patient, **a** longitudinal B-scan showing optic nerve cupping(white arrow), **b** paraxial B-scan revealing the axial myopia, with an axial length of 28.00 mm in the Right eye and 27.00 mm in the left eye

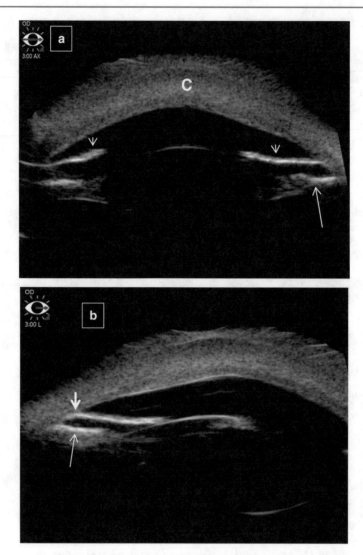

Fig. 8.35 a Axial UBM scan with thickened opaque cornea with greater corneal diameter, thin flat iris with loss of iris pattern (short arrows), thinned stretched–out ciliary body (long arrow), **b** Longitudinal UBM scan exposing the anterior insertion of the iris (thick arrow) with the thin stretched-out ciliary body (thin iris). C: cornea

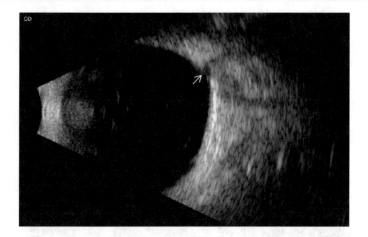

Fig. 8.36 Transverse B-scan of the same patient showing cupping of the optic nerve head with an axial length of 26.00 mm

*Description of the UBM findings in congenital glaucoma emphasized the unique morphology of the ciliary body with massively elongated processes. The stretching is probably due to the enlarging diameter of the eye, creating traction on the zonules attached to a non-enlarging lens. These elongated zonules also cause the greater mobility of the lens in these eyes [14].

*Another interesting finding in these eyes was a thin, stretched-out and rarefied ciliary body [44].

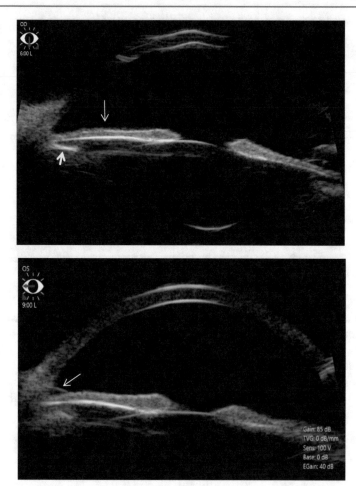

Fig. 8.37 A case of bilateral congenital glaucoma **a** Thinned iris more obvious in the RT eye (thin arrow) and thinned ciliary body(short arrow), **b** with evidence of abnormal angle membrane(white arrow)

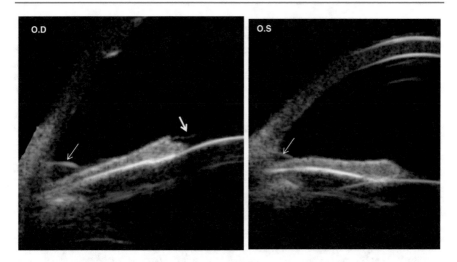

Fig. 8.38 Magnified UBM scans of the previously mentioned patient for more exposure of the abnormal angle membrane in both eyes, i.e. Barkan's membrane, note remnants of persistent pupillary membrane (thick arrow) in O.D

References

1. Ishikawa H, Schuman JS. Anterior segment imaging: ultrasound biomicroscopy. Ophthalmol Clin North Am. 2004;17(1):7.
2. Pavlin CJ, Stuart Foster F. Ultrasound biomicroscopy in glaucoma. Acta Ophthalmol. 1992;70(S204):7–9.
3. Pavlin CJ, Harasiewicz K, Stuart Foster F. Ultrasound biomicroscopy of anterior segment structures in normal and glaucomatous eyes. Am J Ophthalmol. 1992;113(4):381–9.
4. Pavlin CJ, Stuart Foster F. Ultrasound biomicroscopy of the eye. Springer Science & Business Media; 2012.
5. Patwardhan S, et al. Clinical applications of ultrasound biomicroscopy in glaucoma. J Curr Glaucoma Pract. 2007;1(1):30–41.
6. He F, et al. Clinical efficacy of modified partial pars plana vitrectomy combined with phacoemulsification for malignant glaucoma. Eye. 2016;30(8):1094–100.
7. Foreman-Larkin J, Netland PA, Salim S. Clinical management of malignant glaucoma. J Ophthalmol. 2015(2015).
8. Bhende M, et al. Atlas of ophthalmic ultrasound and ultrasound biomicroscopy. JP Medical Ltd.; 2013.
9. Kanadani FN, et al. Ultrasound biomicroscopy in asymmetric pigment dispersion syndrome and pigmentary glaucoma. Arch Ophthalmol. 2006;124(11):1573–6.
10. Golez III E, Latina M. The use of anterior segment imaging after trabeculectomy. Semin Ophthalmol (Taylor & Francis). 2012;27(5–6).
11. Mendrinos E, Mermoud A, Shaarawy T. Nonpenetrating glaucoma surgery. Surv Ophthalmol. 2008;53(6):592–630.
12. Foster PJ, et al. The definition and classification of glaucoma in prevalence surveys. Br J Ophthalmol. 2002;86(2):238–42.
13. Hussein TR, et al. Ultrasound biomicroscopy as a diagnostic tool in infants with primary congenital glaucoma. Clin Ophthalmol (Auckland, NZ). 2014;8:1725.

14. Gupta V, et al. Ultrasound biomicroscopic characteristics of the anterior segment in primary congenital glaucoma. J Am Assoc Pediatric Ophthalmol Strabismus. 2007;11(6):546–50.
15. Sampaolesi R, Caruso R. Ocular echometry in the diagnosis of congenital glaucoma. Arch Ophthalmol. 1982;100:574–7.
16. Adam RS, Pavlin CJ, Ulanski LJ. Ultrasound biomicroscopic analysis of iris profile changes with accommodation in pigmentary glaucoma and relationship to age. Am J Ophthalmol. 2004;138(4):652–4.
17. Yamamoto T, Sakuma T, Kitazawa Y. An ultrasound biomicroscopic study of filtering blebs after mitomycm C trabeculectomy. Ophthalmology. 1995;102(12):1770–6.
18. Greenfield DS, et al. Aqueous misdirection after glaucoma drainage device implantation. Ophthalmology. 1999;106(5):1035–40.
19. Moon K, Kim YC, Kim KS. Ciliary sulcus Ahmed valve implantation. Korean J Ophthalmol. 2007;21(2):127–30.
20. Kumar RS, et al. Confirmation of the presence of uveal effusion in Asian eyes with primary angle closure glaucoma: an ultrasound biomicroscopy study. Arch Ophthalmol. 2008;126 (12):1647–51.
21. Chiou AG-Y, et al. An ultrasound biomicroscopic study of eyes after deep sclerectomy with collagen implant. Ophthalmology. 1998;105(4):746–50.
22. Shi Y, et al. Disease-related and age-related changes of anterior chamber angle structures in patients with primary congenital glaucoma: an in vivo high-frequency ultrasound biomicroscopy-based study. PloS ONE. 2020;15(1):e0227602.
23. Bhatt DC. Ultrasound biomicroscopy: an overview. J Clin Ophthalmol Res. 2014;2(2):115.
24. Panarello SM, et al. Echographic and tomographic evaluation of Molteno and Baerveldt implants in three children. In: Ultrasonography in ophthalmology, vol. XV. Dordrecht: Springer; 1997. p. 219–223
25. Zhang Y, et al. Evaluating subconjunctival bleb function after trabeculectomy using slit-lamp optical coherence tomography and ultrasound biomicroscopy. Chin Med J. 2008;121 (14):1274–9.
26. Aptel F, Dumas S, Denis P. Ultrasound biomicroscopy and optical coherence tomography imaging of filtering blebs after deep sclerectomy with new collagen implant. Eur J Ophthalmol. 2009;19(2):223–30.
27. Avitabile T, et al. Ultrasound-biomicroscopic evaluation of filtering blebs after laser suture lysis trabeculectomy. Ophthalmologica. 1998;212(Suppl. 1):17–21.
28. El Salhy AA, Elseht RM, Al Maria AF, Shalaby SM, Hussein TR. Functional evaluation of the filtering bleb by ultrasound biomicroscopy after trabeculectomy with mitomycin C. Int J Ophthalmol. 2018;11(2):245–50.
29. Mathur R, Gazzard G, Oen F. Malignant glaucoma following needling of a trabeculectomy bleb. Eye. 2002;16(5):667–8.
30. Varma R, et al. Pars plana Baerveldt tube insertion with vitrectomy in glaucomas associated with pseudophakia and aphakia. Am J Ophthalmol. 1995;119(4):401–7.
31. Kumar RS, et al. Prevalence of plateau iris in primary angle closure suspects: an ultrasound biomicroscopy study. Ophthalmology. 2008;115(3):430–4.
32. Jinza K, et al. Relationship between formation of a filtering bleb and an intrascleral aqueous drainage route after trabeculectomy: evaluation using ultrasound biomicroscopy. Ophthalmic Res. 2000;32(5):240–3.
33. Kaushik S, et al. Use of ultrasound biomicroscopy to predict long-term outcome of sub-Tenon needle revision of failed trabeculectomy blebs: a pilot study. Eur J Ophthalmol. 2011;21 (6):700–7.
34. Khairy HA, et al. Ultrasound biomicroscopy in deep sclerectomy. Eye. 2005;19(5):555–60.
35. Yoon K-C, et al. Ultrasound biomicroscopic changes after laser iridotomy or trabeculectomy in angle-closure glaucoma. Korean J Ophthalmol. 2004;18(1):9–14.

36. Marchini G, et al. Ultrasound biomicroscopy and intraocular-pressure-lowering mechanisms of deep sclerectomy with reticulated hyaluronic acid implant. J Cataract Refract Surg. 2001;27(4):507–17.

37. Grigera D, et al. Ultrasound biomicroscopy in eyes with anterior chamber flattening after trabeculectomy. Can J Ophthalmol. 2002;37(1):27–33.

38. Dada T, et al. Ultrasound biomicroscopy in glaucoma. Surv Ophthalmol. 2011;56(5):433–50.

39. Baig NB, Lin AA, Freedman SF. Ultrasound evaluation of glaucoma drainage devices in children. J Am Assoc Pediatric Ophthalmol Strabismus. 2015;19(3):281–4.

40. Carrillo MM, et al. Use of ultrasound biomicroscopy to diagnose Ahmed valve obstruction by iris. Can J Ophthalmol. 2005;40(4):499–501.

41. Sakai H, et al. Uveal effusion in primary angle-closure glaucoma. Ophthalmology. 2005;112 (3):413–9.

42. Kobayashi H, et al. Ultrasound biomicroscopic measurement of development of anterior chamber angle. Br J Ophthalmol. 1999;83(5):559–62.

43. Mannino G, et al. A review of the role of ultrasound biomicroscopy in glaucoma associated with rare diseases of the anterior segment. Clin Ophthalmol (Auckland, NZ). 2016;10:1453.

44. Azuara-Blanco A, et al. Ultrasound biomicroscopy in infantile glaucoma. Ophthalmology. 1997;104(7):1116–9.

45. Shen C-J, Chen Y-Y, Sheu S-J. Treatment course of recurrent malignant glaucoma monitoring by ultrasound biomicroscopy: a report of two cases. Kaohsiung J Med Sci. 2008;24(11):608–13.

46. Shahid H, Salmon JF. Malignant glaucoma: a review of the modern literature. J Ophthalmol. 2012 (2012).

47. Sayed MS, et al. Correlation of echographic and photographic assessment of optic nerve head cupping in children. J Am Assoc Pediatric Ophthalmol Strabismus. 2017;21(5):389–92.

48. Sihota R, et al. Ultrasound biomicroscopy in the subtypes of primary angle closure glaucoma. J Glaucoma. 2005;14(5):387–91.

49. Dusak A, et al. Ultrasound biomicroscopic evaluation of anterior segment cysts as a risk factor for ocular hypertension and closure angle glaucoma. Int J Ophthalmol. 2013;6(4):515.

50. Yoo C, et al. Peripheral anterior synechiae and ultrasound biomicroscopic parameters in angle-closure glaucoma suspects. Korean J Ophthalmol. 2007;21(2):106–10.

51. Marchini G, et al. Ultrasound biomicroscopic and conventional ultrasonographic study of ocular dimensions in primary angle-closure glaucoma. Ophthalmology. 1998;105(11):2091–8.

52. Cronemberger S, et al. New considerations on pupillary block mechanim. Arquivos Brasileiros de Oftalmol. 2010;73(1):9–15.

53. García-Feijoo J, et al. Ultrasound biomicroscopy in Glaucoma. Glaucoma Imaging. 2016:97–121 (Crossref. Web).

Optic Nerve Diseases

9

9.1 Optic Nerve Enlargement

Ocular ultrasonography is very useful in detection of the causes of enlargement of the optic nerve and its sheath. B-scan examination of the optic nerve is usually preformed with medium to low gain settings.

The ideal view for imaging the optic nerve is the vertical transverse approach were the probe is placed temporally at low gain settings. Followed by the longitudinal approach where the probe is placed temporal (close to the limbus and the nerve is displayed at the lower aspect of the scan).

Normal diameter of the retrobulbar optic nerve ranges from 2.2 to 3.3 mm with a mean value of 2.5 mm [1, 23]. Difference of more than 0.5 mm between the two nerves is of significance.

Normal optic nerve reflectivity is low to medium regular internal reflectivity in the anterior one half of the optic nerve with sound attenuation and lower reflectivity in the posterior orbit.

Ultrasound measurement of optic nerve sheath diameter (ONSD) has been validated as an indirect assessment of the increased intracranial tension [2]. Measurements of the optic nerve sheath (ONS) diameter were made with electronic calipers 3 mm behind the posterior scleral surface of the globe [17, 20, 21]. Observational studies in healthy patients confirm that normal ONSD ranges from about 2.2–5 mm [3]. An ONSD of more than 5 mm yields an attractive combination of sensitivity (88%) and specificity (93%) to detect ICP more than 20 cm H_2O [4, 22].

The normal range for optic nerve sheath diameter also has been established for infants and children up to 15 years of age, the range of measured diameter was 2.1–4.3 mm (mean, 3.08 mm) [5]. A sheath diameter of greater than 4 mm in infants under 1 year of age and of greater than 4.5 mm in children age 1–15 years should be considered abnormal [6, 27].

R. Abbas, *Ophthalmic Ultrasonography and Ultrasound Biomicroscopy*,
https://doi.org/10.1007/978-3-030-76979-6_9

Lesions involving the parenchyma such as tumors and inflammations cause homogenous thickening of the nerve. While lesions involving the sheaths such as nerve sheath meningiomas cause irregularly thickened nerves with heterogenous internal echoes [14].

Acquired choroidal folds and optic nerve subarachnoid space enlargement may be signs of idiopathic intracranial pressure elevation [16, 24].

Lesions causing increased subarachnoid fluid, such as pseudotumor cerebri, cause a low reflective widening of the subarachnoid space around the nerve, with 30 degree test may be positive in such cases.

If fluid was seen around the optic nerve, within the sheath, then it was noted as "crescent" or "doughnut" sign positive (Figs. 9.1, 9.2, 9.3, 9.4, 9.5 and 9.6) and it indicated presence of papilledema [7, 29], MRI scan should be requested to find out the cause of papilledema.

30 degree test: The patient fixates in primary gaze (straight ahead position), and the optic nerve pattern is measured anteriorly and posteriorly. The patient's gaze then is directed 30 degree laterally, and the nerve is measured again. The test is based on the premise that when the eye is fixated laterally, the optic nerve sheaths are stretched and the subarachnoid fluid is spread over a larger area. A decrease of the nerve pattern of greater than 10% in lateral gaze, as compared with primary gaze, is considered a positive 30-degree test and thus indicative of increased subarachnoid fluid (Figs. 9.7, 9.8, 9.9 and 9.10).

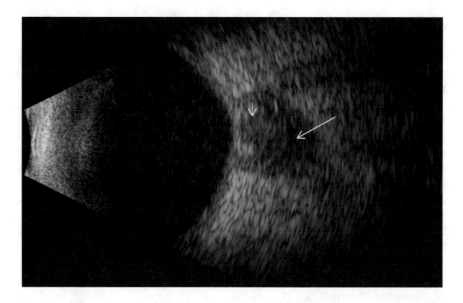

Fig. 9.1 Vertical transverse scan showing marked increase of subarachanoid fluid around the optic nerve forming the doughnut sign, optic nerve (small arrow), the subarachnoid fluid (long arrow)

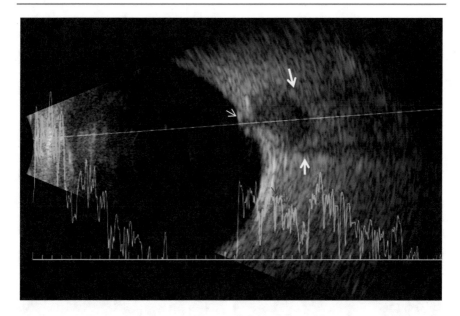

Fig. 9.2 Vertical transverse scan showing elevated optic nerve head (small white arrow) and enlarged optic nerve (thick white arrows) with crescent sign due to increased subarachnoid fluid with irregular internal reflectivity in the superimposed A-scan (red arrows)

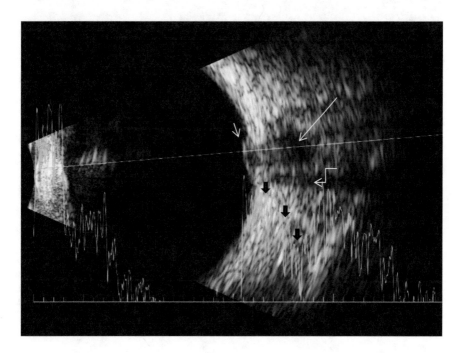

Fig. 9.3 Vertical transverse B-scan showing elevated optic nerve (small arrow) with crescent sign due to increased subarachnoid fluid (long arrow) with sheath widening (elbow arrow), as well as irregular internal reflectivity in A-scan (black arrows)

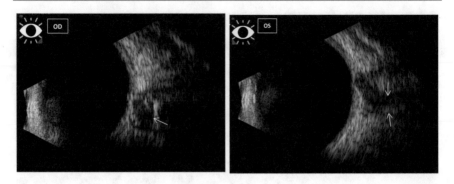

Fig. 9.4 A case of bilateral papilloedema, Bilateral widened optic nerve pattern with doughnut appearance (white arrows) seen in the Right eye (OD) and increased optic nerve sheath (white arrows seen in the LT eye (OS)

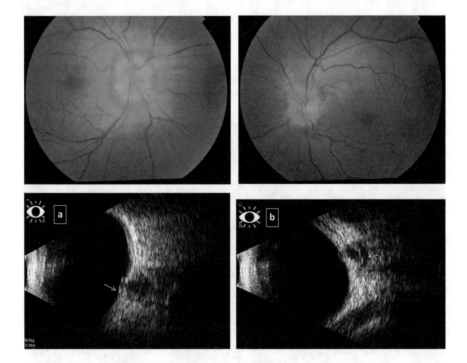

Fig. 9.5 A case of Bilateral papilloedema. The top figures are the fundus photography images of the right and Left eye showing elevated optic nerve head **a** longitudnal scan of the right eye showing elevated optic nerve (white arrow), **b** Vertical transverse scan of the Left eye showing the crescent sign due to increased subarachnoid fluid

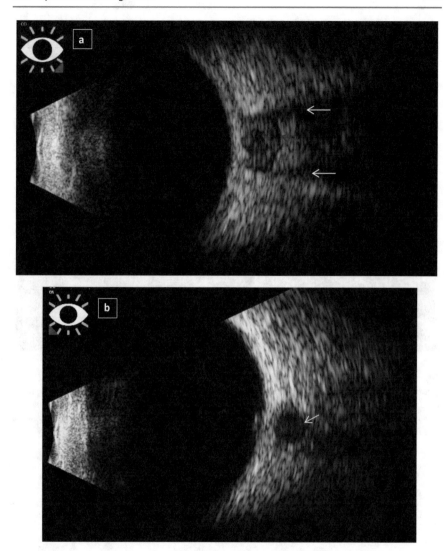

Fig. 9.6 A case with bilateral papilledema **a** Vertical transverse scan of the right eye showing the doughnut appearance (red arrow) with increased optic nerve sheath (white arrows), **b** longitudinal scan of the Lt eye showing doughnut appearance of the optic nerve (arrow)

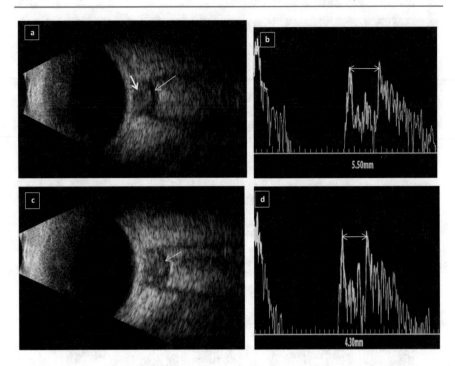

Fig. 9.7 **a** Right eye with subarachnoid fluid (long arrow) around the optic nerve parenchyma (short arrow), **b** measurement of retrobulbar optic nerve diameter while the patient in the primary gaze (straight ahead) with diameter of 5.50 mm. **c** Patient is fixating 30 degree laterally, note the subarachanoid fluid around the optic nerve decreased. **d** Measurement of retrobulbar optic nerve diameter, with diameter of 4.30 mm, denoting positive 30-degree test

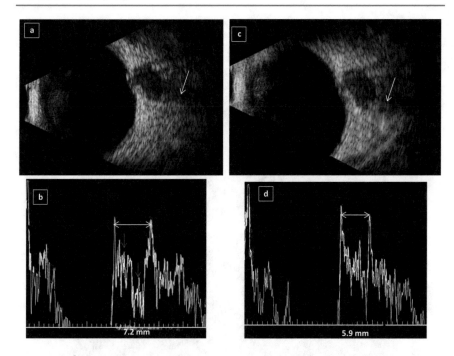

Fig. 9.8 a The Left eye of the same patient in Fig. 9.7, while the patient in primary gaze, showing elevation of optic nerve head with accentuation of the optic nerve sheath (white arrow). **b** Retrobulbar optic nerve diameter (double arrow) with a diameter of 7.2 mm, Note the irregular internal reflectivity on A-scan (red arrows). **c** and **d** Decreased sheath widening (white arrow) when the patient directed his gaze 30 degree laterally. The optic nerve diameter decreased to 5.90 mm, denoting positive 30-degree test

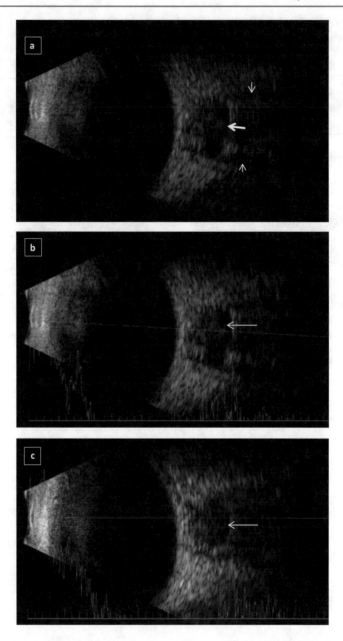

Fig. 9.9 a Vertical transverse B-scan showing widening of the optic nerve with evident crescent sign (white arrow) due to increased subarachnoid fluid with widened optic nerve sheath (short arrows). The same patient with the 30 degree test. **b** Patient in primary gaze with increased subarachnoid fluid around the optic nerve (white arrow) with retrobulbar optic nerve diameter of 7.60 mm. **c** The patient gaze 30 degree laterally causing a decrease of the subarachnoid fluid around the optic nerve (white arrow), and a decrease in the retrobulbar optic nerve diameter to 5.57 mm. Denoting a positive 30 degree test

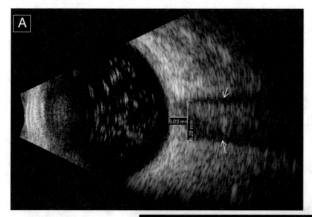

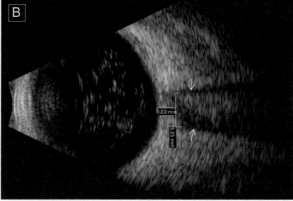

Fig. 9.10 Optic nerve sheath diameter using B-scan calipers **a** while the patient In the primary gaze with 3 mm behind the optic disc, the optic nerve sheath diameter was 6.30 mm. **b** The ONS diameter decreased to 5.35 mm when the patient directed his gaze 30 degrees laterally, denoting a positive 30-degree sign., Note the widened optic nerve sheath in the B-scan (white arrows) in (**a**) compared to the decreased optic nerve sheath (arrows) in (**b**)

9.2   Optic Nerve Lesions

9.2.1   Optic Nerve Glioma

Optic nerve glioma is typically a tumor of childhood [13]. If present in adults, it is more aggressive in nature. It may be associated with neurofibromatosis I. Ultrasound of Optic nerve gliomas seen as smooth fusiform or ovoid thickening of the optic nerve shadow [18]. The internal reflectivity is regular with low to medium reflectivity. In long-standing cases, cystic areas may be seen [25] (Fig. 9.11).

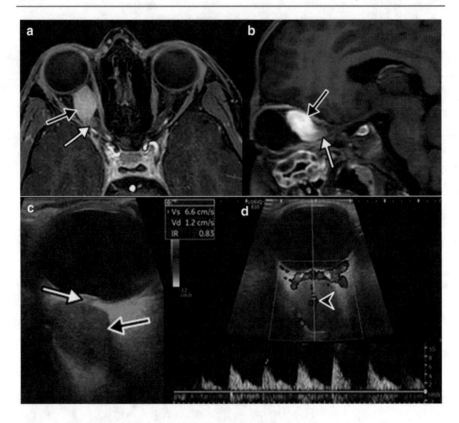

Fig. 9.11 A 10-year-old patient presented with painless progressive loss of vision in the right eye. Magnetic resonance imaging and ultrasound. (Fig A-B) showed a right serpiginous orbital mass (black arrow) in continuity with the optic nerve at both ends (white arrow). Colordoppler flow imaging (CDFI, Fig C) revealed that the central retinal artery (Fig D, black arrowhead) was at the center of the mass, strongly suggesting the diagnosis of optic nerve glioma (ONG). (Chotard, Géraldine, Edgard Farah, and Augustin Lecler. "Color-doppler Flow Imaging Might Help Diagnose Optic Nerve Glioma." Ophthalmology 128.3 (2021): 392) [31]

9.2.2 Melanocytoma

Melanocytoma is a benign and highly pigmented tumor that can emerge almost anywhere in the eye, such as the orbit, iris, ciliary body, choroid, sclera, conjunctiva and the optic disc [12]. The origin of these pigmented lesions is the migration of ectopic melanocytes from the lamina cribosa of the optic nerve head. Melanocytomas are extremely slow-growing tumors. Malignant transformation of a melanocytoma of the optic disc is a highly rare possibility [8].

Melanocytoma is usually a unilateral tumor. The typical papillary lesion is a dark brown or black pigmented tumor, usually located eccentric and on the temporal side. B-scan of the optic nerve melanocytomas are usually mildly elevated with smooth dome shaped lesion, with highly regular internal reflectivity and no internal vascularity (Fig. 9.12) [28].

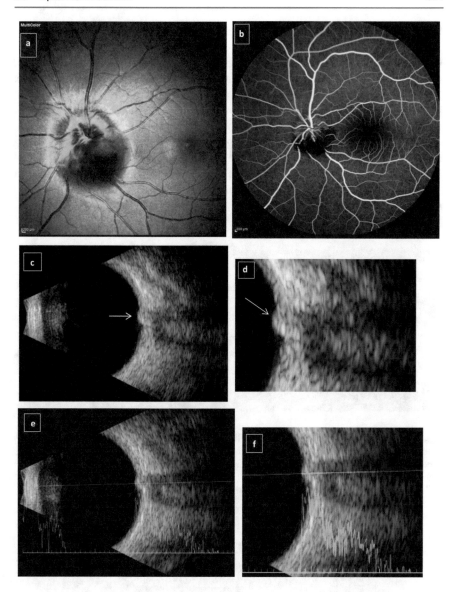

Fig. 9.12 A case of melanocytoma of the optic disc. **a** Fundus photography of the optic nerve head lesion with hypoflourescene seen in (**b**), **c** and **d** Axial scan showing mildly elevated lesion in the temporal edge of the optic nerve head (arrow), **e** and **f** showing the melanocytoma with superimposed A-scan of high amplitude

9.3   Optic Disc Drusen

Optic disc drusen is commonly misdiagnosed as papilledema. Optic nerve head drusen is a calcified lesion that is congenital, originating as a mucoprotein matrix that progressively calcifies over time on the optic nerve itself [9]. It has also been associated with peripapillary retinal neovascularization and hemorrhagic complications in some cases.

Ultrasound is traditionally a good diagnostic method to evaluate patients whom drusen are suspected. Transverse and longitudinal approach often demonstrate the highly reflective echoes of the calcified nodule which persist even in low gain (Figs. 9.13, 9.14 and 9.15). On OCT, eyes with buried drusen can have a decreased retinal nerve fiber layer thickness.

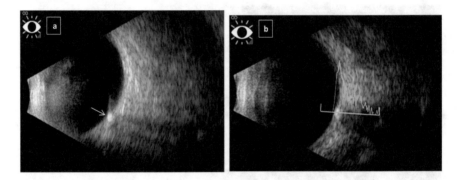

Fig. 9.13 A case of bilateral optic nerve swelling on clinical examination. **a** Right eye with high reflective nodule (white arrow) embedded in the optic nerve head, **b** high amplitude in the superimposed A-scan even at low gain, denoting optic nerve head drusen

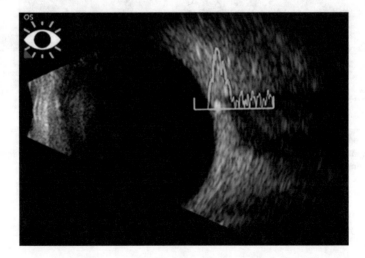

Fig. 9.14 Left eye of the same patient with drusen of high reflectivity embedded in the optic nerve head, with high amplitude in superimposed A-scan

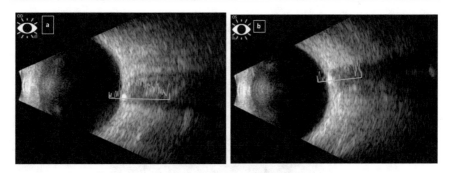

Fig. 9.15 Another case of bilateral Drusen at one edge of the optic nerve head with a nodule of high reflectivity and high reflectivity on the superimposed A-scan

9.4 Optic Nerve Cupping

Optic nerve cupping may be physiological or due to advanced glaucoma. It is best displayed with a vertical transverse B scan and longitudinal scan.

On ultrasound, optic nerve cupping is commonly seen as an excavation at the site of optic nerve entry into the globe. The cup disc ratio must be minimum of 0.5 mm to be detected by ultrasonography (Fig. 9.16) [25, 32, 33].

9.5 Coloboma

Thoroughly explained in the chapter of ocular ultrasonography in pediatrics.

9.5.1 Morning Glory Disc Anomaly

The morning glory anomaly is a rare congenital clinical entity that results from abnormal optic nerve development [10].

The characteristic ophthalmoscopic picture characterized by an enlarged funnel shaped excavated optic disc, at the bottom of which is often a central dot of white fluffy tissue. Surrounding the disc is a wide, grey, elevated annulus of chorioretinal pigment disturbance. The multiple narrow branches of the vessels become visible near the edge of the disc, This disorder was named morning glory syndrome because of the similarity of the ophthalmoscopic picture to the appearance of the flower [10, 19, 30].

*Morning glory syndrome has been associated with other ocular abnormalities such as persistence of primary vitreous and different degrees of retinal detachment [11]. On Ultrasonography is seen as large or deep optic disc excavation (Fig. 9.17).

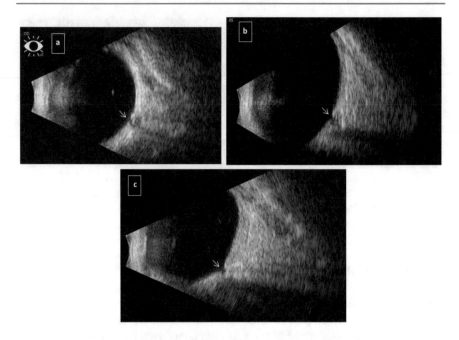

Fig. 9.16 Longitudinal scans of optic nerve head cupping in different patient with variable cup/disc size, starting with small cupping in (**a**) followed by increased cup/disc ratio in (**b** and **c**)

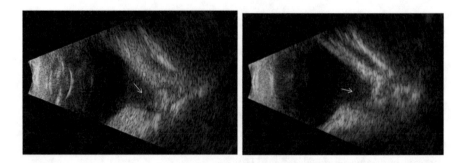

Fig. 9.17 A case of morning glory syndrome. Axial and longitudinal scans revealing a large deep funnel-shaped optic nerve coloboma (white arrows)

References

1. Byrne SF. Ultrasound of the eye and orbit. Mosby Incorporated; 2002.
2. Hassen GW, et al. Accuracy of optic nerve sheath diameter measurement by emergency physicians using bedside ultrasound. J Emerg Med. 2015;48(4):450–7.
3. Agrawal A, et al. Comparison of two techniques to measure optic nerve sheath diameter in patients at risk for increased intracranial pressure. Crit Care Med. 2019;47(6):e495.
4. Kimberly HH, Shah S, Marill K, et al. Correlation of optic nerve sheath diameter with direct measurement of intracranial pressure. Acad Emerg Med. 2008;15(2):201–4.
5. Lystad LD, Hayden BC, Singh AD. Optic nerve disorders. Ultrasound Clin. 2008;3(2):257–66.
6. Le A, et al. Bedside sonographic measurement of optic nerve sheath diameter as a predictor of increased intracranial pressure in children. Ann Emerg Med. 2009;53(6):785–91
7. Bhosale A, Shah VM, Shah PK. Accuracy of crescent sign on ocular ultrasound in diagnosing papilledema. World J Methodol. 2017;7(3):108.
8. Lisker-Cervantes A, et al. Ocular ultrasound findings in optic disk melanocytoma. Revista Mexicana Oftalmol. 2017;91(6):316–20.
9. Rifenburg RP, Williams JJ. Optic nerve head drusen: a case of false-positive papilledema discovered by ocular ultrasound in the emergency department. Crit Ultrasound J. 2010;2 (2):75–6.
10. Haik BG, et al. Retinal detachment in the morning glory anomaly. Ophthalmology. 1984;91 (12):1638–47.
11. Cennamo G, et al. Evaluation of morning glory syndrome with spectral optical coherence tomography and echography. Ophthalmology. 2010;117(6):1269–73.
12. Shields JA, et al. Melanocytoma of the optic disk: a review. Surv Ophthalmol. 2006;51(2):93–104.
13. Dutton JJ. Gliomas of the anterior visual pathway. Surv Ophthalmol. 1994;38(5):427–52.
14. Karolczak-Kulesza M, Rudyk M, Niestrata-Ortiz M. Recommendations for ultrasound examination in ophthalmology. Part II: Orbital ultrasound. J Ultrasonogr. 2018;18(75):349.
15. Watson NJ, Dick AD, Hutchinson CH. A case of sinusitis presenting with sphenocavernous syndrome: discussion of the differential diagnosis. Scott Med J. 1991;36(6):179–80.
16. Lavinsky J, et al. Acquired choroidal folds: a sign of idiopathic intracranial hypertension. Graefe's Arch Clin Exp Ophthalmol. 2007;245(6):883–8.
17. Liu D, et al. Assessment of intracranial pressure with ultrasonographic retrobulbar optic nerve sheath diameter measurement. BMC Neurol. 2017;17(1):1–7.
18. Kerlen CH. B-scan ultrasonography in optic nerve lesions. Doc Ophthalmol. 1982;52(2):317–25.
19. Amador-Patarroyo MJ, Pérez-Rueda MA, Tellez CH. Congenital anomalies of the optic nerve. Saudi J Ophthalmol. 2015;29(1):32–8.
20. Rajajee V, et al. Optic nerve ultrasound for the detection of raised intracranial pressure. Neurocrit Care. 2011;15(3):506–15.
21. Beare NAV, et al. Detection of raised intracranial pressure by ultrasound measurement of optic nerve sheath diameter in African children. Trop Med Int Health. 2008;13(11):1400–04.
22. Chandan G, Matthews N, Clare S. Point of care ultrasound in recognising papilloedema and raised intracranial pressure on the acute medical unit. Clin Med. 2019;19(Suppl 2):110.
23. Neudorfer M, et al. The efficacy of optic nerve ultrasonography for differentiating papilloedema from pseudopapilloedema in eyes with swollen optic discs. Acta Ophthalmol. 2013;91(4):376–80.
24. Nelson ES, Mulugeta L, Myers JG. Microgravity-induced fluid shift and ophthalmic changes. Life. 2014;4(4):621–65.
25. Skalka HW. Ultrasonography of the optic nerve. Neuro-Ophthalmol. 1981;1(4):261–71.
26. Ohno-Matsui K, et al. Evaluation of congenital optic disc pits and optic disc colobomas by swept-source optical coherence tomography. Investig Ophthalmol Visual Sci. 2013;54 (12):7769–78.

27. Steinborn M, et al. High resolution ultrasound and magnetic resonance imaging of the optic nerve and the optic nerve sheath: anatomic correlation and clinical importance. Ultrasound Med Eur J Ultrasound. 2011;32(06):608–13.
28. Salma B, et al. Fortuitously discovered optic nerve tumor: a case report. Asian J Case Rep Surg. 2021:1–4.
29. Shevlin C. Optic nerve sheath ultrasound for the bedside diagnosis of intracranial hypertension: pitfalls and potential. Critical Care Horizons. 2015;1(1):22–30.
30. Hu J. The clinical characteristics and imaging findings of morning glory syndrome. J Huazhong Univ Sci Technol [Med Sci]. 2008;28(4):465.
31. Chotard G, Farah E, Lecler A. Color-doppler flow imaging might help diagnose optic nerve glioma. Ophthalmology. 2021;128(3):392.
32. Darnley-Fisch DA, et al. Contact B-scan echography in the assessment of optic nerve cupping. Am J Ophthalmol. 1990;109(1):55–61.
33. Özen Ö, et al. Evaluation of the optic nerve and scleral-choroidal-retinal layer with ultrasound elastography in glaucoma and physiological optic nerve head cupping. Med Ultrasonogr. 2018;20(1):76–79.

Printed in the United States
by Baker & Taylor Publisher Services